SOAP
for
Orthopedics

Check out the entire SOAP series!

SOAP for Cardiology

SOAP for Emergency Medicine

SOAP for Family Medicine

SOAP for Internal Medicine

SOAP for Obstetrics and Gynecology

SOAP for Neurology

SOAP for Orthopedics

SOAP for Pediatrics

SOAP for Urology

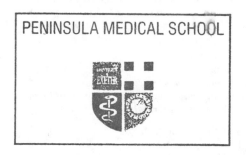

PENINSULA MEDICAL SCHOOL

SOAP
for
Orthopedics

Jonathan R. Gottlieb, MD
Resident, Department of Orthopaedic Surgery
Jackson Memorial Hospital
Miami, Florida

Series Editor
Peter S. Uzelac, MD, FACOG
Assistant Professor
Department of Obstetrics and Gynecology
University of Southern California Keck School of Medicine
Los Angeles, California

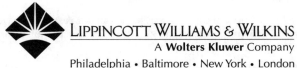

LIPPINCOTT WILLIAMS & WILKINS
A **Wolters Kluwer** Company
Philadelphia • Baltimore • New York • London
Buenos Aires • Hong Kong • Sydney • Tokyo

Acquisitions Editor: Beverly Copland
Development Editor: Selene Steneck
Production Editor: Jennifer Kowalewski
Cover and Interior Designer: Meral Dabcovich
Compositor: International Typesetting and Composition in India
Printer: Sheridan Books in Ann Arbor, MI

351 West Camden Street
Baltimore, MD 21201

530 Walnut Street
Philadelphia, PA 19106

The publisher is not responsible (as a matter of product liability, negligence, or otherwise) for any injury resulting from any material contained herein. This publication
contains information relating to general principles of medical care that should
not be construed as specific instructions for individual patients. Manufacturers'
product information and package inserts should be reviewed for current information, including contraindications, dosages, and precautions.

Printed in the United States of America

Library of Congress Cataloging-in-Publication Data

Gottlieb, Jonathan R.
  SOAP for orthopedics / Jonathan R. Gottlieb.
     p. ; cm. — (SOAP series)
  Includes index.
  ISBN-13: 978-1-4051-0476-0 (pbk. : alk. paper)
  ISBN-10: 1-4051-0476-7 (pbk. : alk. paper) 1. Orthopedics—Handbooks, manuals,
  etc.
  [DNLM: 1. Orthopedic Procedures—Handbooks. WE 39 G686s 2006] I. Title. II.
  Series.
  RD732.5.G68 2006
  616.7—dc22

                                                                    2005010318

*The publishers have made every effort to trace the copyright holders for borrowed mate-
rial. If they have inadvertently overlooked any, they will be pleased to make the necessary arrangements at the first opportunity.*

To purchase additional copies of this book, call our customer service department at
(800) 638-3030 or fax orders to **(301) 824-7390**. International customers should
call **(301) 714-2324**.

Visit Lippincott Williams & Wilkins on the Internet: http://www.LWW.com.
Lippincott Williams & Wilkins customer service representatives are available from
8:30 am to 6:00 pm, EST.

05 06 07 08 09
1 2 3 4 5 6 7 8 9 10

Contents

Reviewers

Prabhat Bhama
Class of 2006
University of Michigan Medical School
Ann Arbor, Michigan

Patrick R. Olson
Class of 2005
University of Utah School of Medicine
Salt Lake City, Utah

Amy Shah
Class of 2006
University of Maryland School of Medicine
Baltimore, Maryland

Esben Vogelius
Class of 2006
UMDNJ — New Jersey Medical School
Newark, New Jersey

To the Reader

Like most medical students, I started my ward experience head down and running, eager to finally make contact with real patients. What I found was a confusing world, completely different from anything I had known during the first two years of medical school. New language, foreign abbreviations, and residents too busy to set my bearings straight: Where would I begin?

Pocket textbooks, offering medical knowledge in a convenient and portable package, seemed to be the logical solution. Unfortunately, I found myself spending valuable time sifting through large amounts of text, often not finding the answer to my question, and in the process, missing out on teaching points during rounds!

I designed the SOAP series to provide medical students and house staff with pocket manuals that truly serve their intended purpose: quick accessibility to the most practical clinical information in a user-friendly format. At the inception of this project, I envisioned all of the benefits the SOAP format would bring to the reader:

• Learning through this model reinforces a thought process that is already familiar to students and residents, facilitating easier long-term retention.

• SOAP promotes good communication between physicians and facilitates the teaching/learning process.

• SOAP puts the emphasis back on the patient's clinical problem and not the diagnosis.

• In the age of managed care, SOAP meets the challenge of providing efficiency while maintaining quality.

• As sound medical-legal practice gains attention in physician training, SOAP emphasizes adherence to a documentation style that leaves little room for potential misinterpretation.

Rather than attempting to summarize the contents of a thousand-page textbook into a miniature form, the SOAP series focuses exclusively on guidance through patient encounters. In a typical use, "finding out where to start" or "refreshing your memory" with SOAP books should be possible in less than a minute. Subjects are always confined to two pages, and the most important points have been highlighted. Topics have been limited to those problems you will most commonly encounter repeatedly during your training and contents are grouped according to the hospital or clinic setting. Facts and figures that are not particularly helpful to surviving life on the wards, such as demographics, pathophysiology, and detailed tables and graphs, have purposely been omitted (such information is best studied in a quiet environment using large and comprehensive texts).

Congratulations on your achievements thus far and I wish you a highly successful medical career!

Peter S. Uzelac, MD, FACOG

Acknowledgements

I would like to thank my parents, Robert and Jo Ann Gottlieb, my fiancée, Nicole, and Christopher Jones, MD for all of their help and support during the writing of this book.

Jonath R. Gottlieb, MD

Abbreviations

ABG	arterial blood gas
AC	acromioclavicular
ACL	anterior cruciate ligament
AP	anteroposterior
aPTT	activated partial thromboplastin time
CBC	complete blood count
CC	coracoclavicular
CFL	calcaneofibular ligament
COX 2	cyclooxygenase 2
CRP	C-reactive protein
CS	compartment syndrome
CT	computed tomography
DDH	developmental dysplasia of the hip
ECG	electrocardiogram
EMG	electromyography
ESR	erythrocyte sedimentation rate
EtOH	alcohol
HIV	human immunodeficiency virus
INR	international normalized ratio
IV	intravenous
LC	lateral compression
LCL	lateral collateral ligament
LCPD	Legg-Calvé-Perthes disease
LMV	lateral meniscal variant
LUCL	lateral ulna collateral ligament
MCL	medial collateral ligament
MI	myocardial infarction
MRI	magnetic resonance imaging
MTP	metatarsophalangeal
MVA	motor vehicle accident
NSAID	nonsteroidal anti-inflammatory drug
OR	operating room
PA	posteroanterior
PCL	posterior cruciate ligament
PO	by mouth
PROM	passive range of motion
pt(s)	patient(s)
PT	prothrombin time
PTT	partial thromboplastin time
ROM	range of motion
RTC	rotator cuff tear
SCFE	slipped capital femoral epiphysis
SPR	superior peroneal retinaculum
TB	tuberculosis

TID	three times daily
WBC	white blood cell
wk(s)	weeks
yr(s)	year(s)

Normal Lab Values

Blood, Plasma, Serum

Aminotransferase, alanine (ALT, SGPT)	0–35 U/L
Aminotransferase, aspartate (AST, SGOT)	0–35 U/L
Ammonia, plasma	40–80 µg/dL
Amylase, serum	0–130 U/L
Antistreptolysin O titer	Less than 150 units
Bicarbonate, serum	23–28 meq/L
Bilirubin, serum	
Total	0.3–1.2 mg/dL
Direct	0–0.3 mg/dL
Blood gases, arterial (room air)	
Po_2	80–100 mm Hg
Pco_2	35–45 mm Hg
pH	7.38–7.44
Calcium, serum	9–10.5 mg/dL
Carbon dioxide content, serum	23–28 meq/L
Chloride, serum	98–106 meq/L
Cholesterol, total, plasma	150–199 mg/dL (desirable)
Cholesterol, low-density lipoprotein (LDL), plasma	≤130 mg/dL (desirable)
Cholesterol, high-density lipoprotein (HDL), plasma	≥40 mg/dL (desirable)
Complement, serum	
C3	55–120 mg/dL
Total	37–55 U/mL
Copper, serum	70–155 µg/dL
Creatine kinase, serum	30–170 U/L
Creatinine, serum	0.7–1.3 mg/dL
Ethanol, blood	<50 mg/dL
Fibrinogen, plasma	150–350 mg/dL
Folate, red cell	160–855 ng/mL
Folate, serum	2.5–20 ng/mL
Glucose, plasma	
Fasting	70–105 mg/dL
2 hours postprandial	<140 mg/dL
Iron, serum	60–160 µg/dL
Iron binding capacity, serum	250–460 µg/dL
Lactate dehydrogenase, serum	60–100 U/L
Lactic acid, venous blood	6–16 mg/dL
Lead, blood	<40 µg/dL
Lipase, serum	<95 U/L
Magnesium, serum	1.5–2.4 mg/dL

Manganese, serum	0.3–0.9 ng/mL
Methylmalonic acid, serum	150–370 nmol/L
Osmolality plasma	275–295 mOsm/kg H_2O
Phosphatase, acid, serum	0.5–5.5 U/L
Phosphatase, alkaline, serum	36–92 U/L
Phosphorus, inorganic, serum	3–4.5 mg/dL
Potassium, serum	3.5–5 meq/L
Protein, serum	
Total	6.0–7.8 g/dL
Albumin	3.5–5.5 g/dL
Globulins	2.5–3.5 g/dL
$Alpha_1$	0.2–0.4 g/dL
$Alpha_2$	0.5–0.9 g/dL
Beta	0.6–1.1 g/dL
Gamma	0.7–1.7 g/dL
Rheumatoid factor	<40 U/mL
Sodium, serum	136–145 meq/L
Triglycerides	<250 mg/dL (desirable)
Urea nitrogen, serum	8–20 mg/dL
Uric acid, serum	2.5–8 mg/dL
Vitamin B_{12}, serum	200–800 pg/mL

Cerebrospinal Fluid

Cell count	0–5 cells/µL
Glucose (less than 40% of simultaneous plasma concentration is abnormal)	40–80 mg/dL
Protein	15–60 mg/dL
Pressure (opening)	70–200 cm H_2O

Endocrine

Adrenocorticotropin (ACTH)	9–52 pg/mL
Aldosterone, serum	
Supine	2–5 ng/dL
Standing	7–20 ng/dL
Aldosterone, urine	5–19 µg/24 h
Cortisol	
Serum 8 AM	8–20 µg/dL
5 PM	3–13 µg/dL
1 h after cosyntropin usually ≥8 µg/dL above baseline	>18 µg/dL
overnight suppression test	<5 µg/dL
Urine free cortisol	<90 µg/24 h
Estradiol, serum	
Male	10–30 pg/mL

Female
  Cycle day 1–10   50–100 pmol/L
  Cycle day 11–20   50–200 pmol/L
  Cycle day 21–30   70–150 pmol/L

Female	
Cycle day 1–10	50–100 pmol/L
Cycle day 11–20	50–200 pmol/L
Cycle day 21–30	70–150 pmol/L
Estriol, urine	>12 mg/24 h
Follicle-stimulating hormone, serum	
Male (adult)	5–15 mU/mL
Female	
Follicular or luteal phase	5–20 mU/mL
Midcycle peak	30–50 mU/mL
Postmenopausal	>35 mU/mL
Insulin, serum (fasting)	5–20 mU/L
17-Ketosteroids, urine	
Male	8–22 mg/24 h
Female	Up to 15 µg/24 h
Luteinizing hormone, serum	
Male	3–15 mU/mL (3–15 U/L)
Female	
Follicular or luteal phase	5–22 mU/mL
Midcycle peak	30–250 mU/mL
Postmenopausal	>30 mU/mL
Parathyroid hormone, serum	10–65 pg/mL
Progesterone	
Luteal	3–30 ng/mL
Follicular	<1 ng/mL
Prolactin, serum	
Male	<15 ng/mL
Female	<20 ng/mL
Testosterone, serum	
Adult male	300–1200 ng/dL
Female	20–75 ng/dL
Thyroid function tests (normal ranges vary)	
Thyroid iodine (^{131}I) uptake	10% to 30% of administered dose at 24 h
Thyroid-stimulating hormone (TSH)	0.5–5.0 µU/mL
Thyroxine (T4), serum	
Total	5–12 pg/dL
Free	0.9–2.4 ng/dL
Free T4 index	4–11
Triiodothyronine, resin (T3)	25%–35%
Triiodothyronine, serum (T3)	70–195 ng/dL
Vitamin D	
1,25-Dihydroxy, serum	25–65 pg/mL
25-Hydroxy, serum	15–80 ng/mL

Gastrointestinal

Fecal urobilinogen	40–280 mg/24 h
Gastrin, serum	0–180 pg/mL
Lactose tolerance test	
Increase in plasma glucose	>15 mg/dL
Lipase, ascitic fluid	<200 U/L
Secretin-cholecystokinin pancreatic function	>80 meq/L of HCO_3 in at least 1 specimen collected over 1 h
Stool fat	<5 g/d on a 100-g fat diet
Stool nitrogen	<2 g/d
Stool weight	<200 g/d

Hematology

Activated partial thromboplastin time	25–35 s
Bleeding time	<10 min
Coagulation factors, plasma	
Factor I	150–350 mg/dL
Factor II	60%–150% of normal
Factor V	60%–150% of normal
Factor VII	60%–150% of normal
Factor VIII	60%–150% of normal
Factor IX	60%–150% of normal
Factor X	60%–150% of normal
Factor XI	60%–150% of normal
Factor XII	60%–150% of normal
Erythrocyte count	4.2–5.9 million cells/μL
Erythropoietin	<30 mU/mL
D-dimer	<0.5 μg/mL
Ferritin, serum	15–200 ng/mL
Glucose-6-phosphate dehydrogenase, blood	5–15 U/g Hgb
Haptoglobin, serum	50–150 mg/dL
Hematocrit	
Male	41%–51%
Female	36%–47%
Hemoglobin, blood	
Male	14–17 g/dL
Female	12–16 g/dL
Hemoglobin, plasma	0.5–5 mg/dL
Leukocyte alkaline phosphatase	15–40 mg of phosphorus liberated/h per 10^{10} cells
Score	13–130/100 polymorphonuclear neutrophils and band forms

Leukocyte count	
Nonblacks	4000–10,000/µL
Blacks	3500–10,000/µL
Lymphocytes	
$CD4^+$ cell count	640–1175/µL
$CD8^+$ cell count	335–875/µL
CD4/CD8 ratio	1.0–4.0
Mean corpuscular hemoglobin (MCH)	28–32 pg
Mean corpuscular hemoglobin concentration (MCHC)	32–36 g/dL
Mean corpuscular volume (MCV)	80–100 fL
Platelet count	150,000–350,000/µL
Protein C activity, plasma	67%–I 31%
Protein C resistance	2.2–2.6
Protein S activity, plasma	82%–144%
Prothrombin time	11–13 s
Reticulocyte count	0.5%–1.5% of erythrocytes
Absolute	23,000–90,000 cells/µL
Schilling's test (oral administration of radioactive cobalamin–labeled vitamin B_{12})	8.5%–28% excreted in urine per 24–48 h
Sedimentation rate, erythrocyte (Westergren)	
Male	0–15 mm/h
Female	0–20 mm/h
Volume, blood	
Plasma	
Male	25–44 mL/kg body weight
Female	28–43 mL/kg body weight
Erythrocyte	
Male	25–35 mL/kg body weight
Female	20–30 mL/kg body weight

Urine

Amino acids	200–400 mg/24 h
Amylase	6.5–48.1 U/h
Calcium	100–300 mg/d on unrestricted diet
Chloride	80–250 meq/d (varies with intake)
Copper	0–100 µg/24 h
Creatine	
Male	4–40 mg/24 h
Female	0–100 mg/24 h
Creatinine	15–25 mg/kg per 24 h

Creatinine clearance	90–140 mL/min
Osmolality	38–1400 mOsm/kg H_2O
Phosphate, tubular resorption	79%–94% (0.79–0.94) of filtered load
Potassium	25–100 meq/24 h (varies with intake)
Protein	<100 mg/24 h
Sodium	100–260 meq/24 h (varies with intake)
Uric acid	250–750 mg/24 h (varies with diet)
Urobilinogen	0.05–2.5 mg/24 h

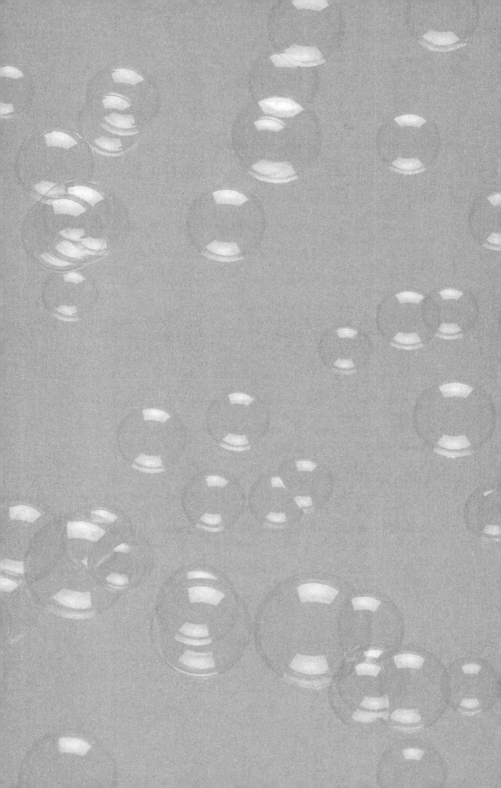

S **What was the cause of the injury?**
With the rare exception of pathologic fractures, acetabular fractures are invariably the result of high-energy trauma such as motor vehicle crash or a fall from a great height.
- Crush injuries can cause significant soft tissue injury and lead to wound healing problems after surgery.

O **Perform physical exam starting with the ABCs**
The orthopedic assessment follows the trauma team's evaluation of the pt.
- Associated injuries can involve any organ system given the high-energy nature of these fractures.

Ensure that the skin is intact.
Are the leg lengths equal?
- Acetabular fractures can result in proximal femoral migration into the pelvis.

Is there an expanding hematoma?
- This is suggestive of an arterial injury or large venous rupture.

Does the pt have symmetric pulses in the feet?
- Asymmetric pulses suggest an arterial injury or spasm and must be worked up further.

Are the sensory and motor functions intact in the leg?
- Contusions to nerves or stretch injuries (neurapraxias) may temporarily (for many months) compromise sensation and function.
  - More severe nerve injuries may result in permanent loss of function.

Is the pelvis stable to compression? Is there blood at the urethral meatus or rectum?
- Injuries to these structures are less common than with other pelvic ring fractures but may occur.
- Assess that the four extremities are without deformity, have full range of motion, and are nontender.
- Acetabular injuries are painful and distract from other injuries.

Obtain plain x-rays of the pelvis

All acetabular fractures are initially evaluated with an anteroposterior view of the pelvis followed by Judet views.
- Judet views are 45-degree oblique x-rays of the pelvis and are needed to classify the fracture (obturator and iliac obliques).

Obtain CT scan to further evaluate the fracture pattern
Plain films may miss small, non-displaced fracture lines or incarcerated fragments within the joint.
  - 3-D reconstructions of the acetabulum are useful in preoperative planning.

Acetabular fracture

Diagnosis is radiographic, and pattern and displacement of the fracture dictate treatment.

The acetabulum is the point in the innominate bone where the ilium, ischium, and pubis come together; in children, this area consists of the triradiate cartilage.

The acetabulum and innominate bone can be divided into anterior and posterior columns.

- The anterior column consists of the anterior wall of the acetabulum, anterior iliac wing, pelvic brim, and superior pubic ramus.
- The posterior column consists of the posterior wall of the acetabulum and the ischium.

Classification is based on Letournel: 5 simple and 5 associated

Five simple fractures are:

- Posterior wall	- Posterior column
- Anterior wall	- Anterior column
- Transverse	

Five associated (complex) fractures are:

- Associated posterior column and posterior wall
- Associated transverse and posterior wall
- T shaped
- Associated anterior and posterior hemitransverse
- Both column

Plan to open, reduce, and fix

Contraindications to surgery include infection, severe osteoporosis, and severe soft tissue or visceral injuries.

- These pts can be treated with distal femoral skeletal traction for 6 wks followed by remaining non–weight bearing for an additional 6 wks (or until callus is visible on plain films).

Non-displaced fractures and those that do not involve the weight-bearing surface of the acetabulum are managed with non–weight bearing and total hip precautions (limited flexion, internal rotation, abduction).

- The weight-bearing surface of the acetabulum is the superior 10 mm.

Surgery should ideally be performed several days after the injury

This allows the bleeding around the fracture to subside.

Choice of surgical approach is based on fracture pattern.

- Kocher-Langenbeck is most commonly used as it gives access to the posterior wall and column (most common fracture locations).
- Ilioinguinal gives overall best exposure to the anterior column.
- Extended iliofemoral allows access to both columns but has significant complications (prolonged recumbency and ectopic bone).

S
What are the chief complaints?
Can range from discomfort with activity in the area of the tendon that is relieved by rest to severe pain and inability to plantar flex the foot

Was there an acute injury?
Achilles tendon ruptures are acutely painful events that may be precipitated by chronic pain but are often without previous discomfort.
- Most occur during athletic events.
- Tendinosis and peritendinosis of the Achilles tendon are more chronic.

O
Perform physical exam
Is the pt able to walk on the affected leg?
- Weight bearing is exceedingly difficult after Achilles tendon ruptures but will be possible (though painful) with peritendinitis, tendinosis, or a partial rupture.
  - Tendinosis is often minimally painful, though.
Where is the pain localized?
- Pain is noted in the distal Achilles tendon several cm proximal to its insertion.
Is the heel swollen?
- Swelling is acute and severe in ruptures.
- Also significant in calcaneus fractures, though

Can the pt perform a single heel rise?
- Usually not possible with rupture of the tendon
Is Thompson's test positive?
- If squeezing the calf does not elicit passive plantar flexion, the tendon is ruptured.

Is the pain exacerbated by resisted plantar flexion?
- Even with complete rupture the foot can often be plantar flexed because of the intact peroneal and deep posterior compartment tendons.
Is there a palpable gap in the tendon?
- Consistent with a complete rupture
Are there palpable nodules or a mass in an intact tendon?
- Consistent with tendinosis

Obtain x-rays of the ankle
These usually are nonspecific.
- Calcifications in the tendon and calcaneal osteophytes may be noted in chronic conditions.

Use ultrasound to confirm a suspected rupture
Ultrasound is a safe and inexpensive method to confirm the presence of a ruptured tendon.

Use MRI in equivocal cases or to confirm chronic pathologic process
Should not be required to diagnose a rupture but is useful for demonstrating inflammatory and/or degenerative changes

Achilles Tendon Injury

The Achilles tendon is the terminal portion of the gastrocnemius and soleus muscles, which coalesce and insert into the posterior calcaneus.

- The tendon has a vascular watershed area 2–6 cm proximal to the insertion due to reliance on proximal and distal blood supply.
- This is the area most prone to inflammation and rupture.
- Risk factors for the development of injury to the Achilles tendon include increase in duration or intensity of training, rapid return to activity after prolonged inactivity, poor running form, or running on uneven surfaces.

Injuries can be divided based on area of pathology and chronicity

Peritendinitis is inflammation of the peritenon only.

- Pain and tenderness are noted at the distal area of the tendon and are aggravated by activity and mitigated by rest.

Tendinosis is the chronic result of repetitive microtrauma to the tendon that results in the classic, painless nodule in the distal tendon.

- The process begins with peritendinitis that develops into scarring and adhesions to the tendon, ultimately compromising blood supply and resulting in scarring of the tendon.
- The condition may be painless but acute inflammation can develop.

Achilles tendon ruptures can be complete or partial.

- Partial tears occur in young, athletic pts and can be clinically difficult to discern from a severe strain; MRI can help.
  - The lateral aspect of the tendon is usually involved.
- Complete ruptures are seen in intermittently active, middle-aged males.
  - The classic pop followed by pain and plantar flexion weakness with a positive Thompson's sign is nearly diagnostic.

 Manage peritendinitis conservatively

Rest, ice, stretching, and administration of NSAIDs are the cornerstones of initial treatment.

If conservative methods fail after several months, surgical lysis of adhesions can be performed, excising the scarred peritenon.

Consider a nonoperative trial as well

Short-term casting followed by the protocol for peritendinitis should be continued for 6 months.

- Augment with a controlled active motion walker or orthosis to correct any hindfoot deformity.
  - If this fails, debride the peritenon and tendon.
  - Areas of necrotic tendon or scarring are excised; if the defect is large, use an Achilles flap or the flexor digitorum longus or plantaris tendon to reinforce the defect.

Consider surgical repair

Surgical repair of the ruptured Achilles tendon is more effective than casting.

Small defects in partial tears can be managed with therapy; large partial tears and complete rupture should be primarily repaired whenever possible.

- The rerupture rate is 10 times higher in pts treated without surgery.

S

How did the injury occur?
Usually the result of direct trauma, such as blow to the shoulder with a blunt instrument or a fall onto the shoulder
- Can also be the result of indirect trauma, such as a fall on an outstretched arm
  - Indirect forces force the humeral head up into the acromion, stretching the ligaments of the acromioclavicular (AC) joint complex.

Is the injury acute or chronic?
Determination of chronicity and previous injuries is important in determining management.
- Weightlifters and athletes involved in contact sports are predisposed to chronic AC joint injuries refractory to conservative management.

O

Perform physical exam
What is the position of the arm?
- The arm is usually held waist level and supported with the other arm.
- If it is fixed in internal rotation, be suspicious of a posterior shoulder (glenohumeral) dislocation.

Evaluate skin for abrasions, lacerations, or tenting.
- The subcutaneous nature of the clavicle and AC joint increases the likelihood of open injuries.
- Tightly tented skin may necrose several days later, creating an open wound.
- Significant swelling and discoloration may be seen acutely.
  - An expanding hematoma suggests a vascular injury.

Point tenderness over the AC joint is usually present.
Gross instability of the clavicle usually cannot be elicited in the acute setting due to pain and guarding.
- After the initial symptoms have resolved or in chronic settings, anteroposterior (AP) and vertical motion at the AC joint can be seen.

Neurovascular competence of the extremity should be assessed.
- The subclavian artery and brachial plexus run just deep to the clavicle medially and can be injured.
- Pulses and capillary refill should be assessed and compared with the contralateral side.
- Confirm both sensation and motor function of the axillary, musculocutaneous, median, radial, and ulnar nerves.

Obtain x-rays
A trauma shoulder series (AP, axillary, and scapular Y views) with a Zanca view (tube is angled 15 degrees cephalic) is needed to diagnose and classify the injury.
- Associated fractures (especially distal one-third clavicle) or dislocations are seen.
- CT and MRI are not needed.

Acromioclavicular joint injury

Anatomy: the AC joint is a diarthrodial joint consisting of the distal clavicle and the medial facet of the acromion.
- The joint is stabilized by a capsule and capsular ligaments.
- Stability of the joint in the AP plane is conferred by the AC ligaments.
  - Most significant of these ligaments is the superior AC ligament.
- Vertical stability is maintained by the coracoclavicular (CC) ligaments, the conoid and trapezoid.
  - Both ligaments must be disrupted for complete superior displacement of the clavicle to occur.

Diagnosis and classification are made on the basis of radiographic findings.
- Type I: Isolated sprain of AC ligament (no displacement)
- Type II: AC ligaments disrupted but CC intact (<50% vertical displacement of clavicle)
- Type III: AC and CC disrupted (complete disassociation of AC joint)
- Type IV: Type III with clavicle buttonholed through trapezius (posterior displacement of clavicle is confirmed on axillary x-ray)
- Type V: Type III with greater than 100% elevation of clavicle
  - The result of deltoid and trapezius avulsion from distal clavicle
- Type VI: Type III with clavicle inferior to corocoid

Plan is dependent of severity of injury, chronicity, and functional demands

Type I injuries, when seen acutely, are stable.
- Ice, elevation, NSAIDs, and short-term sling for comfort with return to activity as tolerated.
- Chronic AC injuries should also initially be managed conservatively but this often fails, necessitating distal clavicle resection with early return to activity.

Acute type II injuries can also be managed conservatively, though some physicians prefer short-term immobilization to ensure the injury does not convert to a type III.
- Degenerative changes are more common with type II injuries than type I.
- Chronic type II AC injuries are managed as type I chronic injuries.

Type III injury management is debatable.
- Some physicians manage these injuries as type I/II or use a harness.
- Many suggest that athletes should undergo surgical fixation.
- Surgical procedures include internal fixation of the joint, CC ligament reconstruction, resection of the distal clavicle, and transfer of the corocoid process with its muscle attachments to the clavicle.
- No study has ever proven which treatment is superior.

Pts with type IV injuries should undergo open reduction, repair of the deltotrapezial fascia, and reconstruction of the CC ligament.
- The coracoacromial ligament is sacrificed and used for the CC reconstruction.

Type V and VI injuries should undergo open reduction with ligamentous reconstruction and fascial repair.
- Resection of the distal clavicle reduces likelihood of AC joint arthritis.

S

How did the injury occur?
Anterior cruciate ligament (ACL) tears are usually the result of a noncontact, pivoting injury.
  • More often seen in younger, active individuals
  • Pts will generally say that they felt a "pop" followed by severe pain in the knee.

What are the pt's functional demands?
The pt's age, activity level, and general health are important in determining the treatment protocol.

O

Perform physical exam
Significant swelling from hemarthrosis is noted almost immediately.
Often, pain and swelling limit one's ability to perform the physical exam.
Range of motion (ROM) and areas of tenderness should be assessed first.
Key tests for the ACL include:
  • Lachman's test: flex the knee to 30 degrees and pull the tibia forward, assessing laxity and for an endpoint.
    ◆ Most sensitive test for ACL tear
  • Anterior drawer: flex the knee to 90 degrees and pull the tibia forward.
  • Pivot shift: while placing valgus and internal rotation stresses on the knee, flex the knee.
    ◆ When the knee is extended, a pop will be felt as the tibia reduces.
The posterior cruciate ligament (PCL), lateral collateral ligament (LCL), and medial collateral ligament (MCL) should also be assessed.
All knees with ACL tears should also be evaluated for meniscal tears.
  • Tenderness to palpation of the medial and lateral joint lines
  • Mechanical block to ROM
  • Positive McMurray's test

Evaluate x-rays of the knee
Three views of the knee: anteroposterior, lateral, and sunrise
  • Findings seen with ACL tears include avulsion of the tibial spine and the Segund sign.
  • The Segund sign is a small capsular avulsion of the lateral tibia.
  • Changes consistent with degenerative joint disease (Fairbank's changes) should also be noted as ACL repairs in degenerative knees fare poorly.
  • Squaring of the femoral condyles, peaking of the tibial spines, and joint space narrowing are seen in degenerative knees.

Use MRI to confirm the diagnosis
The history and physical exam are the cornerstones of diagnosis, but MRI is useful in confirming the diagnosis as well as locating any other injury.

Anterior Cruciate Ligament Tear

The ACL originates on the posteromedial lateral femoral condyle and inserts on the tibia just anterior and between the intercondylar eminences.

- It consists of two bundles of fibers: anteromedial (tight in flexion) and posterolateral (tight in extension).
- The main function of the ACL is to prevent anterior translation of the tibia with respect to the femur.
- The blood supply of the ACL comes from branches of the middle geniculate artery.

ACL tears are most commonly seen in young athletes, with the incidence being greater in females than males.

- Females are felt to be more prone to these injuries due to smaller femoral notches and ligaments and different mechanics of the knee.
- In adults, tears of the ACL tend to be midsubstance, whereas children often have avulsion injuries.

 Consider a reconstruction

The decision whether or not to repair a torn ACL in an adult is based on several factors: the pt's functional level, demands, and injury pattern.

- ACL tears with concomitant rupture of a collateral ligament (LCL or MCL) or repairable meniscal tears should be reconstructed.
- Isolated ACL tears in competitive athletes should undergo reconstruction.
- Isolated ACL tears in sedentary individuals should generally be managed non-operatively.

Nonoperative management consists of aggressive strengthening and range-of-motion exercises about the knee.

Pts undergoing ACL reconstruction should continue physical therapy preoperatively until full flexion and extension are reached.

- Knee stiffness after ACL reconstruction is most commonly seen when surgery is performed prior to full ROM.
- Arthrofibrosis, often requiring arthroscopic debridement, is also associated with surgery performed too acutely.

Reconstruction is usually performed with arthroscopic assistance.

- Autograft versus allograft reconstruction using bone-patella, tendon-bone, hamstring, or quadriceps is based mainly on the surgeon's preference.

Plan for early and aggressive postoperative therapy

Immediate use of continuous passive motion machines, early weight bearing, and closed-chain concentric exercises are used in most rehabilitation schemes.

S **How does the pt describe the pain?**

Chief complaint will be pain out of proportion to injury or event and severe pain with movement of limb.

Obtain history of event (if an acute event occurred)
Most compartment syndromes develop after a high-energy trauma, such as motor vehicle accident or fall.
- Also associated with snake bites, drug overdoses, overzealous hydration in burn pts, and IV infiltrates

If no event is elicited in history, consider vascular causes
Leakage from vascular access vessels, revascularization procedures, spontaneous bleeds in coagulopathic pts

 Perform physical exam
The affected limb will usually be swollen and the fascial compartments tight.
The signs of an acute compartment syndrome include:
- Pain out of proportion to injury or event; it is always worse with passive stretching of the muscle.
- Paresthesias will develop after 1 hr of ischemia time.
- Pallor
- Paralysis
- Pulselessness

Pain out of proportion is the key!
- By the time the other signs of compartment syndrome develop, irreversible damage may already be occurring.

- In addition, compartment syndromes can occur without the development of the other physical exam findings classically described.
- Loss of distal pulses and pallor do not usually occur unless there is an arterial injury or the compartment pressures are nearly that of the tissue pressures.

The disappearance of pain does not signify that the compartment syndrome is resolving.
- Disappearance of pain is indicative of the onset of irreversible nerve damage.
- Once painlessness or paralysis has developed, minimal recovery of function is possible.

If compartment syndrome is suspected or the pt cannot provide subjective information, measure compartment pressures
Pts who have pain with tight compartments or obtunded pts in whom the diagnosis is suspected should have objective measurements of their compartment pressures.
- This is can be performed using an arterial line connected to an 18-gauge needle.
- The line should be zeroed after each compartment is measured.

- If the pressure within any compartment is within 20 mm Hg of the diastolic pressure, the diagnosis of acute compartment syndrome is assigned.

- If the compartment pressures are rising and are near this critical level, the pressures should be remeasured every 1–2 hrs.

Order relevant lab tests and/or imaging indicated by the cause of syndrome onset
Addressing the compartment syndrome will be of no benefit if the cause is ignored.
- Fractures should be evaluated radiographically.
- Medical causes should be properly worked up.
- Vascular injuries should be evaluated in an expeditious manner.

Acute compartment syndrome

Acute compartment syndrome develops when the pressure in the fascial compartments exceeds that of perfusion.

It can occur in any part of the body where fascial compartments are found.
- Most commonly found in the leg and forearm

By both convention and experimental results, compartment syndrome is defined by an intracompartmental pressure that is within 20 mm Hg of the diastolic pressure.
- Tissue edema from trauma, cell destruction, or reperfusion or expansile hematomas all increase the pressure in the affected compartment.
- As the pressure increases, the low pressure capillary drainage system backs up, increasing the pressure in the arterioles.
- Tissue perfusion then decreases, ischemia develops, and muscles and nerves begin to sustain irreversible damage.

Skeletal muscle can survive up to 4 hrs of total ischemia with no irreversible changes.
- After 6 hrs, variable irreversible changes are noted.
- By 8 hrs of total ischemia, the muscle is completely destroyed.

Peripheral nerves will sustain only neurapraxic damage after 4 hrs of total ischemia.
- By 8 hrs, the nerve will be rendered irreversibly nonfunctional.
- Ischemic contractures and loss of sensation can render limbs completely useless.

P **Acute compartment syndromes must be managed aggressively and quickly**

Consider medical management

Medical management has limited applications.

Most practical is the liberal use of ice to cool the tissues and possibly diminish swelling.

Muscles and nerves that have sustained cool versus warm ischemia have better survivability.

This is most useful when reperfusion cannot be performed in a timely fashion.

Any coagulopathy, poisoning, or other medical cause should be addressed prior to surgery.

Consider surgical management

Surgical management is the gold standard.

Decompression of hematoma
Repair or ligation of bleeding vessels

Decompressive fasciotomies should extend the full length of the compartment.

External fixation should be used to stabilize any long bone fractures.

Follow renal function closely

In cases of delayed or missed diagnosis, renal function must be closely monitored.

Significant myonecrosis will result in myoglobinuria and, potentially, renal damage.
- Diuresis should be promoted with copious IV fluids to eliminate the protein.
- Aggressive debridement of dead muscle also helps reduce the myoglobin load faced by the kidneys.

S **Obtain the history of the event**
When did the injury occur? What was the pt doing at the time?
- Usually an indirect (twisting) mechanism

Did the pt hear or feel a pop?
- Suggestive of a fracture or ligament rupture

Is weight bearing possible?
Where is the pain localized?
Is there pain anywhere else?
Are there any abnormal sensations or areas of numbness?
- Neurovascular injuries are uncommon but do occur with ankle fractures.

Obtain a detailed medical and social history
Prior injuries
Previous surgery on the foot or ankle
General medical condition
- Diabetes
- Vascular disease
- Immunocompromised states

Smoking
- Associated with increased risk of infection, nonunion

Living conditions
- Indigent pts may have compliance issues.
- Consider stairs, whether help is available at home

 Obtain radiographs
Three views each of foot and ankle
Two views of tibia/fibula and knee
- High-energy injuries associated with syndesmotic disruption and fractures at proximal fibula may occur.
- Pattern and mechanism of injury important in determining reduction maneuver and surgical options.
- Evaluate for any other abnormalities, especially in the foot.

Perform physical exam
General: Evaluate other extremities, spine, pelvis for any overlooked injuries.
Knee/leg: Pain, range of motion (ROM), swelling
- Possible ligamentous injury or fracture

Foot/ankle: Swelling
- Is the foot too swollen to cast or splint?
- May a compartment syndrome be developing?

Skin/soft tissue envelope
- Is this an open fracture?

Neurovascular status
- Though rare, vascular compromise warrants further investigation.
- Nerve injuries tend to be neurapraxias, which usually resolve over time (up to several months).

ROM of feet and toes

Address preoperative labs/medical clearance
Otherwise healthy young adults usually need minimal medical workups.

Bimalleolar ankle fracture
Diagnosis is suspected based on history and confirmed radiographically
Can be classified based on mechanism of injury and fracture pattern

- Lauge-Hansen: Four injury patterns describe 95% of ankle fractures
  - Supination-adduction
  - Supination–external rotation (most common)
  - Pronation-abduction
  - Pronation–external rotation
- Weber: based on level of fibular fracture (higher level denotes higher energy injury)
  - A: below level of syndesmosis
  - B: at level of syndesmosis
  - C: above level of syndesmosis

Bimalleolar equivalent is lateral malleolus fracture with deltoid ligament rupture.

Trimalleolar fracture also includes a fracture of the posterior tibial plafond.

Initial management usually involves immobilization
Open fractures emergently to operating room (within 6 hrs)
Vascular compromise or compartment syndromes are also emergent.
Closed fractures should be reduced after adequate analgesia and placed in a U splint (long leg preferable).
Non–weight bearing on the affected side
Ice and elevation
Monitor swelling and neurovascular condition

Definitive management should be operative

Outcomes with surgical fixation of bimalleolar ankle fractures are markedly better than with closed (even near-anatomic) reduction and casting.

- Open reduction, internal fixation when swelling permits (earlier is better)
Postoperative: non–weight bearing for 6 wks in short leg cast
  - Weight bearing is then advanced in a walking cast.

Consider exceptions to surgery
Medically unstable pts

Pts with poor healing potential (advanced vascular disease, diabetics)

Pts with active bacterial infections

S **What are the presenting complaints (according to parents or pediatrician)?**
Babies born with brachial plexus injuries demonstrate abnormal posturing and/or diminished movement of the affected arm, depending on level of injury.

What risk factors does the baby have for the injury?
Anything that makes delivery more difficult increases the likelihood of injury.
- Consider size (large), prolonged labor, multiparous pregnancy, fetal distress, breech delivery, maternal diabetes.
  - Fetal distress may render the child hypotonic and thus more susceptible to stretch injuries.

O **Perform physical exam**
Obviously, newborns will not respond to commands and cooperate during an exam.
- Observation for spontaneous shoulder, arm, wrist, and finger movements
- Stimulation of neonatal reflexes (such as Moro and Votja) is done to provoke movement.

Is Horner's syndrome present?
- Interruption of the sympathetic chain indicates a preganglionic lesion (injury to the nerve is actually an avulsion from the spinal cord) that will not heal.
- Other signs concerning for a preganglionic lesion include absence of rotator cuff function, scapular winging, rhomboid, and/or latissimus dorsi function.

Imaging studies are usually not required
There is no indication for plain films other than to rule out a fracture or dislocation.
- The risk factors for obstetric brachial plexus injuries are the same as those for clavicle fractures.

MRI and CT myelography have been used to determine whether the lesion was a cord avulsion or extraforaminal (pre- or postganglionic).

Electromyelograms and nerve conduction velocities have proven unreliable is assessing likelihood of recovery.
- Most clinicians rely on the physical exam and progression of function for determination of level and management.

Obstetric brachial plexus injury

Occur in 0.1% to 4% of all live births

Mechanism of injury is stretching of the brachial plexus during delivery, resulting in traction injury to the nerves.
- The usual scenario involves a shoulder dystocia whereby after delivery of fetal head the shoulder gets stuck under the pubis symphysis. Continued traction on head in the presence of immobile body results in stretching of brachial plexus nerves.

Determining the level of injury is essential for assessing the likelihood of recovery, and this is based on the physical exam findings.

Consider the anatomy:
- Brachial plexus receives contributions from the anterior spinal nerve roots of C5 to T1.
  - 20% to 25% of cords also receive a contribution from C4.
- Upper trunk consists of C5 and C6, middle trunk C7, and lower trunk C8 and T1.
  - Each trunk has anterior and posterior bifurcations called divisions.

Different injury patterns are described:
- Upper trunk (C5-C6; Erb's palsy) injuries are most common but have the best prognosis.
  - Arm is held in classic "waiter's tip" position and affected muscles are the rotator cuff, deltoid, elbow flexors, and wrist/hand dorsiflexors.
- Lower trunk (C8-T1; Klumpke's palsy) are less common and have a worse prognosis, especially when associated with preganglionic lesions.
  - Wrist flexors and hand intrinsics are affected; Horner's syndrome (ptosis, meiosis, anhydrosis) seen if lesion is preganglionic (it usually is).
- Total plexus (C5-T1) injuries carry the worst prognosis and the arm is flaccid.

Multiple classification schemes have been proposed but are of limited usefulness.

- Biceps function and Horner's syndrome appear to be the best predictors of functional outcome.
  - Both the absence of biceps function at 6 months and the presence of Horner's syndrome carry a poor prognosis.

 Management initially should be conservative

90% of cases will resolve with no intervention and motor function may continue to improve for 18 months to 2 yrs.
- Physical therapy for 3 months to maintain range of motion of the shoulder, elbow, wrist, and fingers is the hallmark of early treatment.
- Biceps function and Horner's syndrome determine the next step.
  - If the biceps returns, continue physical therapy until age 2 yrs.
  - If it does not return and Horner's is present, reconstruction of the brachial plexus is undertaken.
  - If biceps does not return but Horner's is not present, continue 3 more months of therapy.
  - If still no biceps at 6 months, do brachial plexus reconstruction.

If signs of recovery are seen in first 2 months of life, function will generally be normal.
- If recovery is delayed for longer than 3 months, the likelihood of recovery diminishes and permanent strength and motion deficits are likely.

With plexus reconstructions, other surgeries are sometimes needed

These include contracture releases, muscle/tendon transfers, and various osteotomies

S **What are the chief complaints?**

Presenting complaints can be quite variable.
- May include pain, paresthesias, and muscle weakness in various patterns and to different degrees
- Classic complaint is radicular pain with radiation to trapezius and periscapular region.
- Symptoms are often described as changing with position of the head.
  - Worse pain with "tilting the head back"
- Is the pt having difficulty with ambulation or any changes in bladder and bowel function?
  - These symptoms are more consistent with cord compression.

How long have symptoms been present?

Compression of the exiting nerve root may be the result of an acute event (disk herniation after trauma) or from degenerative changes seen with spondylosis.
- Treatment differs for more diffuse, degenerative disorders.

O **Perform physical exam**

Up to 70% of pts with radiculopathy have motor and/or reflex disturbances.

Specific findings are noted with each root radiculopathy.
- C1 and C2 radiculopathies are quite rare: typical manifestations are occipital headaches, jaw pain; no motor deficit.
- C3 radiculopathy is more common: presents with posterior neck pain and headaches that are clinically similar to tension headaches; no motor deficit.
- C4 radiculopathy: neck and trapezius pain; sometimes numbness at neck and shoulders; no motor deficit.
- C5 radiculopathy: classic findings are pain and/or numbness of shoulders and posterior arm; deltoid muscle is weakened.
  - Rotator cuff and elbow flexors may be weakened.
  - Biceps reflex is mediated by C5 and may also be diminished.
- C6 radiculopathy: pain or disturbances in sensation from neck to biceps and down to tips of thumb and index finger; wrist extensors are weakened.
  - Rotator cuff, triceps, and thumb extensors may be weakened.
  - Brachioradialis reflex often diminished
- C7 radiculopathy: pain or sensory abnormalities from back of neck, posterior arm, and extending into middle finger; triceps muscle weak.
  - Wrist flexors, finger extensors often weakened
  - Triceps reflex often absent
- C8 radiculopathy: pain is uncommon; symptoms are usually seen distal to wrist and present like ulnar nerve neuropathy.
  - Interossei are weakened.
  - This rare entity should elicit investigation for ulnar nerve pathology.

Obtain plain x-rays despite the fact that they have a limited value in cervical radiculopathy

Anteroposterior, lateral, oblique, and open mouth views should be evaluated for degenerative or other pathologic processes in the spine.
- In general, films should not be obtained until 6 wks of conservative therapy has failed.

MRI is better than CT for evaluation of soft tissue pathologic lesions
Disk herniations and changes within the roots themselves are better viewed with
MRI than CT, although CT myelograms allow better delineation of osseous and
calcific pathologic lesions.

Determine cause of radiculopathy
Acute radiculopathies are usually due to disk herniations; chronic changes usually
lead to more insidious onset of symptoms.

- The differential diagnosis for radiculopathy includes tumors, peripheral nerve
entrapment syndromes, myelopathy, and thoracic outlet syndrome.

Cervical radiculopathy
Diagnosis is clinical and based on sensory and/or motor changes in sclerotomal
distribution.
- Any cause of root compression will give radicular symptoms.
- Disk herniation, ligamentous hypertrophy, degenerative changes, infection, and
even chemical irritation can compress exiting nerve roots.

- C6 and C7 radiculopathies are the most common.

- Disk herniations and spondylosis are responsible for 90% of cases.

- Approximately 90% of the time radiculopathy resolves without surgery.

Attempt nonoperative treatment first
If the deficit is worsening or debilitating (inability to extend wrist, for example), the
conservative management is surgical.

- In addition, if the cause of the radiculopathy is infectious, tumor, or secondary
to trauma, surgical intervention may be warranted.

Nonsurgical modalities are numerous:
- Short-term immobilization (soft collar for less than 2 wks)
- Home traction (literature reveals conflicting results)
- Physical therapy
- Pharmacologic intervention (NSAIDs, muscle relaxants; avoid oral steroids)
- Epidural steroids are often effective in relieving radicular symptoms.

Indications for surgery are specific
Symptoms persisting beyond 6 wks
Debilitating motor weakness
Worsening neurologic deficit
Associated spinal instability

S
What is the pt's primary complaint?
A wide range and variety of complaints are possible.
- In some pts cord compression is completely asymptomatic.
- Pain can range from isolated neck pain to diffuse upper extremity discomfort.
- Paresthesias are common and are often diffuse in the upper extremity
- Weakness in upper extremity, lower extremity, or both may be present.
- Often the first complaint is difficulty with gait and balance.
- Bowel and bladder dysfunction are rare.

Increasing difficulty with daily activities involving fine motor coordination, such as buttoning, zippering, and writing, are common complaints.

How long have symptoms been present?
Symptoms have usually been present for several years, and periods of improvement and worsening are usually described; an acute onset suggests another diagnosis (trauma, tumor).

Are any risk factors present?
Risk factors include:
- Frequent lifting
- History of excessive driving
- Cigarette smoking
  - Cigarette smoking is also associated with worse clinical outcomes and more serious perioperative complications.

O
Perform a physical exam
Assess ambulation and the ability of the pt to walk on heels and toes.
Neck: examine for range of motion (ROM), tenderness, and worsening of symptoms with motion.
- ROM is generally decreased, especially extension.
- Decreased and painful extension suggests frank cord compression and increased risk of iatrogenic injury during intubation.
Full neurologic exam of upper and lower extremities should be performed.
- Strength of muscles representing all testable nerve roots
- Wasting of shoulder girdle musculature and the hand intrinsics should be noted.
- Sensation to light touch, vibration, and pinprick along all dermatomes
- Reflexes usually reveal hyperreflexia (with concomitant nerve root compression, reflexes may be diminished).
- Long tract signs may be present (clonus, inverted radial reflex, and Babinski's and Hoffmann's tests).
- Cranial nerve dysfunction suggests a possible brainstem lesion.

Begin radiographic evaluation with plain films
Anteroposterior (AP), lateral, oblique, and flexion-extension films should be obtained.
- Common findings include disk space narrowing, endplate sclerosis, and osteophytosis.
- Oblique views show foraminal narrowing.
- Lateral view demonstrates sagittal alignment and canal size.
- AP view useful for evaluation of scoliotic deformity.

Obtain an MRI

This is indicated in pts in greater than 2–3 months of neck pain, neurologic findings, or worsening symptomatology.

- Demonstrates the extent of soft tissue pathologic processes (disks, ligaments, etc.)
- Also useful for evaluation of cord (myelomalacia, presence of syrinx or tumor) and the space available for cord (normally 17 mm; <13 mm is abnormal)

Order additional tests as indicated

CT gives better definition of the posterior longitudinal ligament, which can become ossified.

Electrodiagnostic testing may be useful when neurologic disease or severe neuropathy is in the differential.

Cervical spondylotic myelopathy

A slowly progressing process of degeneration in the spine

- Disks, facet joints, and uncovertebral joints degenerate.
- Results in disk bulging, hypertrophy of ligaments, and osteophyte development
- Space available for cord diminishes, as does the area where nerve roots exit
- Instability and compensatory subluxations allow the process to progress.
- Ultimately, cord (and often exiting nerve roots) is compressed and symptoms worsen.

- Ossification of the posterior longitudinal ligament, most often seen in Asians, gives same clinical picture even in the absence of spondylotic changes.

Conservative modalities are usually the first step in management

Observe pts who have no signs or symptoms of myelopathy, regardless of radiographic findings.

- However, if the canal compromise is so severe that even a low-energy injury may result in cord compression, surgery is warranted even if the pt is without symptoms.

In cases of mild myelopathy (such as those with no weakness but only gait disturbances), conservative treatment may be continued.

- This includes the use of NSAIDs, moist heat, physical therapy, soft collars

Consider surgery based on the clinical extent of myelopathy

Surgery for neck pain only is poorly efficacious.

Surgical options are broad and include:

- Anterior discectomy/corpectomy and fusion (generally the preferred technique)
- Laminectomy: has fallen out of favor due to instability
- Laminoplasty: Very useful, but may limit ROM postoperatively

Both laminoplasty and anterior decompression and fusion are effective 90% of the time.

The procedure of choice is based on both clinical findings and surgeon comfort with each procedure.

- For example, laminoplasty should not be performed in kyphotic pts.
- Pts who require multilevel corpectomies should not be treated with the anterior approach due to the increased rate of pseudarthrosis.

What has the family or caregiver observed?
Clubfoot is a problem that is glaringly obvious to the family and the practitioner.
- The foot is markedly deformed and malrotated.
- Other disorders distressing to the parents may also be present (described below).

Review medical history
How old is the child?

- Early (immediate) management tends to give better results.

- Families must understand that delays in treatment will change the outcome.
Does the child have any medical problems that may limit treatment options?
Does the child have any other disorders associated with clubfoot?
- Streeter's dysplasia (constriction band syndrome leading to truncated/amputated extremities)
- Diastrophic dwarfism
- Arthrogryposis (especially distal arthrogryposis syndrome)
- Spina bifida (or other dysraphism)
- Other neuromuscular or paralytic disorders

Is there a family history of clubfoot?

One fourth of pts with congenital clubfoot have a positive family history.

Did the child have any early amniocentesis?
Recent evidence has linked amniocentesis at 11–12 wks with the development of clubfoot.

 Perform full-body physical exam
General: evaluate for any dysmorphic features.
- It is essential to look for any malformations or abnormalities that may suggest an associated syndrome or medical issue that must be addressed.
Spine: look for hairy patches or dimples suggestive of dysraphism.
Extremities: evaluate for symmetry, range of motion (ROM), muscle tone.
- Findings in associated disorders may be discrete, especially early in life.
- Calf on affected side is generally smaller in diameter than that on unaffected side (if unilateral).
Neurologic: full neurologic exam is essential due to associated disorders.

Foot: forefoot is in adduction and supination; the hindfoot is in equinus and varus.
- ROM and flexibility of deformity have important prognostic implications.

Obtain studies of the foot
Standard x-rays should be evaluated: simulated weight-bearing anteroposterior (AP) and lateral views of the foot
- The value of the films is questionable due to the mostly cartilaginous nature of young bones.
- Normally, the angle between the talus and calcaneus is >35 degrees on the lateral x-ray.
  ◆ This is decreased in clubfoot.
- The talocalcaneal angle is normally 20–40 degrees on the AP.
  ◆ In clubfoot it is less than 20 degrees.

On both views, increased "parallelism" is noted between the talus and calcaneus.

No lab tests are needed to diagnose clubfoot
If any of the associated conditions require further evaluation, the proper lab tests should be done.

Clubfoot (congenital talipes equinovarus)

Incidence varies with race, but all show 2:1 male preponderance.
Bilateral disease occurs in 50% of cases.

Progression will be relentless if untreated but pain is usually minimal.
Diagnosis is clinical with radiographic evaluation.
Several classification schemes have been developed but are not particularly useful.
Etiology is poorly understood but recent theories suggest a disorder in muscle
   development.
   • Whether this is the result of genetics, environment, or a combination is unclear.

 Assessment of need for further workup should be done
Given the high association with other disorders (including genetic), any additional
   suspected abnormalities should be evaluated.

Plan for immediate intervention. Timely management is essential.
Initially, nonsurgical intervention is suggested.
Casting methods have demonstrated improving outcomes.

   • The Ponsetti casting method has a reported success rate of 90%.

   • Following correction, the child is to be placed in a Denis Browne bar full time
     until he or she is able to stand, and then at night only.
   • Splinting may be continued until school age.
   • Most children treated with casting require an Achilles tendon release to correct
     equines.
   • In addition, 25% will require a tibialis anterior tendon transfer later to correct
     the development of forefoot adduction and supination deformities.
Physiotherapy and continuous passive motion are used in Europe with equally
   impressive reported success rates, but this has not been adopted in the U.S.

Consider surgery
Surgery is required in recalcitrant cases.

Soft tissue transfer with tendon lengthenings is performed at 6–9 months when
   non-surgical interventions have failed.

Releases are as limited as possible to correct the deformity.
   • Posteromedial release is the procedure favored by most surgeons.
Postoperative immobilization and return to activity is variable among authors.
Older children require bony correction and have worse outcomes than infants.
   • Children aged 3–10 yrs may benefit from aggressive osteotomy.
   • Older children require a triple arthrodesis.

Surgical risks are significant and should be discussed with parents or caregiver
These include growth arrest, over- or undercorrection, wound healing problems, and
   vascular injuries

The posterior tibial artery may be the only vessel to the foot (absent dorsalis pedis).

S

Does the pt complain of any changes in sensation?
Pain and paresthesias (usually on palmar-radial aspect of hand)
  - Often worse at night
  - Exacerbated by extreme flexion/extension (as in driving) or repetitive hand motions

Have the symptoms progressed?
Usually a gradual progression occurs in entrapment, though acute compressions can occur after trauma (distal radius fracture classic) and these are surgical emergencies.

Does the pt complain of clumsiness?
Pts frequently complain of dropping things.
  - Can be related to changes in sensation
  - Also associated with weakness of the thenar muscles

Does the pt have any risk factors for carpal tunnel syndrome?
These are numerous, but include:

- Acromegaly	- Diabetes	- Alcoholism
- Gout	- Pregnancy	- Raynaud's disease
- Rheumatoid arthritis		

  - Occupational (repetitive wrist movements such as typing, piano playing, manual labor)

O

Perform physical exam
A variety of clinical tests are used; positive test results in parenthesis.
  - Phalen's test: wrists are flexed for 60 seconds (paresthesias)
  - Tinel's test: tapping over carpal tunnel (tingling in radial fingers)
  - Carpal tunnel compression test: squeeze carpal tunnel by hand (paresthesias)
Motor: bulk and strength of thenar muscles
  - Atrophy and weakness of thenar muscles is noted in advanced disease.
Sensation: subjective and objective measures of sensation are important.
  - Light touch (Semmes-Weinstein monofilaments): assess slowly adapting fibers.
  - Static two-point discrimination: assess slowly adapting fibers (suggests advanced median nerve dysfunction).
  - Moving two-point discrimination: assess quickly adapting fibers (suggests advanced median nerve dysfunction).

Order x-rays
Plain x-rays are usually not helpful but they should be evaluated to rule out any pathologic or posttraumatic changes.

Consider EMG
EMG is the gold standard for evaluation of nerve compression.

Evaluates sensory and motor nerve conduction velocities and latencies
  - However, it is operator dependent.
  - Also, normal EMG findings have been described in up to 20% of pts with surgically documented compression.
  - Comparison with the contralateral side is essential.

Consider proximal or systemic causes
Cervical root compression, thoracic outlet syndrome, ligament of Struthers
Metabolic or degenerative neurologic disorders

Carpal Tunnel Syndrome

The most common compressive neuropathy in the upper extremity

- Essentially a chronic compartment syndrome of the carpal tunnel
- Direct measurements of pressures usually reveal pressures greater than 25 mm Hg.
- The roof of the compartment is the transverse carpal ligament.
- Associated risk factors described above result in pathologic synovium.
  - ◆ This synovium is the most common cause of idiopathic carpal tunnel syndrome.
  - ◆ Fibrosis, edema, lymphocytes, and amyloid deposits are seen.

It is essential to differentiate acute from chronic carpal tunnel syndrome.

- If there is any question, carpal tunnel pressures must be measured.
- Irreversible median nerve damage will result from missing an acute carpal tunnel syndrome.

Nonsurgical treatment should be tried first

Splinting of wrist in neutral (decompresses and removes stretch from nerve)

NSAIDs (reduce inflammation)

Diuretics (reduce edema within compartment)

Ergonomically correct workstations and tools

Physical therapy

Steroid injections are effective initially in 80% of pts

After 1 yr, only 22% still have relief of symptoms.

Pts who do best from steroid injections are those with less than 1 yr of symptoms, mild paresthesias, and no weakness.

If conservative methods fail, surgical decompression should be performed

Either open or endoscopic decompressions can be utilized.

- Long-term results of the two procedures are equal.
- Rehabilitation is accelerated by about 2 wks with endoscopic releases.
  - ◆ Failure to completely release the transverse carpal ligament is the most common complication of endoscopic releases.

Surgeon experience is the most important factor in success of the surgery.

Repeat carpal tunnel releases are less effective

Only 25% pts will have complete resolution of symptoms with a re-release.

- Pts who do best with repeat releases are those with nocturnal symptoms, short incisions, and relief of symptoms with steroid injections.
- Success of repeat releases is no greater in cases where the transverse carpal ligament was incompletely released initially.

S **Was the pt referred by another physician?**
In the U.S., pediatricians evaluate the hips of newborns and report any abnormalities they encounter to an orthopedist.

The birth history (gestational age, type of delivery, complications, position) should be discussed.

Does the child have any risk factors for developmental dysplasia of the hip (DDH)?
The congenital form is associated with several risk factors:
- Breech positioning   - First born
- Female   - Positive family history

Does the child have any disorder that may be associated with hip dysplasia?
These are numerous and include:
- Neurologic disorders (myelomeningocele)
- Myopathies (arthrogryposis)
- Syndromes (Larsen's syndrome)
- Connective tissue diseases (Ehlers-Danlos syndrome)

O **Perform general physical exam**
The child should be seen in the nursery and the hips evaluated last.
Evaluate for conditions associated with DDH.
- Generalized ligamentous laxity
- Abnormal muscle tone
- Hairy patches or discolorations in the midline of the back (consistent with dysraphism)
- Torticollis or metatarsus adductus ("packaging problems")
- Dislocations or contractures of any other joints

Lower extremities should be closely scrutinized
Asymmetric skin folds in the gluteal or inguinal region suggest DDH.
Leg lengths should be equal (inequality suggests DDH).
- Allis' test (asymmetry in femoral lengths versus hip dislocation)
  - If both hips are dislocated, Allis' test is unreliable.
Hip range of motion and any mechanical obstruction noted
- Abduction is often limited in DDH but not until infant is several months old.
- Soft clicks without evidence of instability are considered normal variants.
Barlow's and Ortolani's tests determine stability of the hip.
- Barlow's test determines whether hip is defined as subluxable (femoral head remains within the acetabulum) or dislocatable.
  - Performed by adducting and depressing of the femur to dislocate a dislocatable hip.
- Ortolani's test reduces a dislocated hip with elevation and abduction of the femur.
- Barlow's and Ortolani's tests become negative after 3 months as soft tissue contractures develop.

Plain x-rays should be obtained but are often unreliable
Normal films may be found in children with clinically unstable hips.
AP pelvis should be scrutinized to evaluate for teratologic hip dislocations as well as any pelvic, spinal, or femoral abnormality.
- Teratologic hips are defined as those with a pseudoacetabulum at birth.

Radiographs are most helpful in children older than 3 months.

- At that point, the presence of delayed ossification and acetabular dysplasia may be visible.

Ultrasound can be used to confirm dislocatable hips
Dynamic ultrasound is highly sensitive.

- Ultrasound can also be used to confirm concentric reduction.

Developmental dysplasia of the hip
Developmental dysplasia of the hip (DDH) has replaced the old term "congenital dysplasia or dislocation of the hip."

- Congenital dislocatable or subluxable hips is the most common subtype.
- The term refers to any disorder that results in abnormalities in development and growth of the hip, including the proximal femur and/or acetabulum.

1/1000 children is born with a dislocated hip.
1/100 is born with a dysplastic or subluxable hip.

The left hip is dysplastic 60% of the time, the right 20%, and both 20%.

The goal of treatment is to obtain and maintain a concentric reduction
This is the only way to prevent the later development of degenerative joint disease.

Most infants (<6 months) <u>without</u> teratologic dysplasia can be treated with a Pavlik harness
Concentric reduction of the hip must be confirmed with radiographs or ultrasound.
The legs are placed in 100 degrees of flexion and mild abduction.
After 2 wks, the hips are re-evaluated for stability.
If the hips are stable at 2 wks, the harness is weaned and follow-up x-rays are obtained to ensure that the dysplasia is resolving.

Neonates with subluxed hips at birth are not placed into a harness unless the subluxation has not resolved by 3 wks of age.

If the Pavlik fails, the hip cannot be reduced, or there is teratologic dysplasia:
Attempts at closed reduction and spica casting can be made under anesthesia, though if the Pavlik has failed after 3 wks, this should not be attempted.
Open reduction is generally only performed in infants with teratologic dysplasia but may also be warranted with irreducible dislocations or unstable hips.

- The main risk of open and closed reduction is femoral head osteonecrosis.

- This occurs because of direct injury to or impingement of the posterosuperior retinacular branch of the medial femoral circumflex artery

Children older than 6 months generally require surgical correction

S

What are the chief complaints?
Diabetic foot infections can range from a mild ulcer to painless gas gangrene in a pt with neuropathy.

Has the pt had a diabetic ulcer before?
The most sensitive predictor of future ulceration or infection is a history of an ulcer.

O

Perform physical exam
Diabetic pts should be followed and evaluated routinely by their internist and endocrinologist, who should perform a full physical exam.
- The orthopedist is also responsible for determining whether the pt is systemically ill.

Orthopedic diabetic foot exam starts with observation.
- Is the skin intact or are there any ulcers (and how deep are they)?
- Is the skin red or shiny? Is hair present? Are the nails dysmorphic?
- Is there an abscess or area of fluctuance that may require drainage?
- Is there any subcutaneous air that may represent gas gangrene?
- Have any amputations been performed?

Is sensation intact to light touch, pinprick, and two-point discrimination?
- Diminished sensation in the plantar foot is often the first sign of diabetic neuropathy and an at-risk foot.

Are the pulses palpable?
- Nonpalpable pulses suggest concomitant vascular disease.
  - The dorsalis pedis pulse is usually the last pulse lost.

Obtain x-rays of the foot
Three views of the foot are needed (anteroposterior, lateral, and oblique).
Evaluate for signs of osteomyelitis, fractures, gas gangrene, or a Charcot foot.
- Signs of osteomyelitis include periosteal reaction, sequestrum, or involucrum.
- Gas gangrene is a surgical emergency; pts may not yet be systemically ill but treatment should not be delayed.
- Charcot feet will show diffuse osteopenia, multiple fractures and dislocations, and midfoot collapse early with later sclerosis and malunion.

Send labs and cultures
CBC, comprehensive metabolic profile, HbA$_{1C}$
- Total protein level > 6.2, serum albumin > 3.5, and total lymphocyte count > 1500 are the levels needed for optimal healing.

Ensure the pt will heal the infection or ulcer
Further workup of healing potential is required prior to intervention.
- Transcutaneous oxygen tension (TcPO$_2$) should be evaluated by hyperbaric medicine; a level of 30 mm Hg is required for tissue to heal.
- Arterial doppler pressures of 40 mm Hg in the toes or 70 mm Hg in the ankle are required for ulcers or amputations to heal.
- Ankle brachial indices and pulse volume recordings are also utilized to determine the healing capacity of the foot.
- CT, triple phase bone scan, and MRI can also be used if the diagnosis is in question.

Diabetic foot ulcer
Classification scheme used is Wagner's
- Grade 0: No open lesions but foot at risk
- Grade 1: Superficial ulcer
- Grade 2: Deep ulcer with extension to bone, joint, or tendon
- Grade 3: Deep abscess or osteomyelitis
- Grade 4: Gangrene of the toes or forefoot
- Grade 5: Gangrene of entire foot

Ulcers which are not yet infected often become so.

- ½ pts who present with a diabetic foot infection will have an infection in the opposite foot within 1½ yrs.
- The most common infectious organisms are *Staph* species, *Streptococcus* species, and gram (-) bacteria.

  - Anaerobic bacteria are cultured in ⅓ infected diabetic feet.

 Treat infections aggressively
Local cellulitis may be treated with IV followed then oral antibiotics while abscesses and osteomyelitis require debridement.
- Antipseudomonal penicillin until symptoms improve followed with a fluoro-quinolone is often effective for cellulitis.
- Osteomyelitis should be treated with 6 wks of parenteral antibiotic.

Treat ulcers based on their clinical grade
Grade 0: Serial exams of foot with well-fitted shoes and insoles
Grade 1: Local debridement then total contact cast (re-evaluated every 2 wks)
Grade 2: Local debridement in OR with total contact cast (changed every week)
Grade 3: Resection of infected bone and casting with biweekly wound checks
Grade 4: Local amputation versus revascularization by vascular surgery
Grade 5: Major (below or above knee) amputation

Total contact casts should be continued until the ulcer has healed

S   **What are the complaints?**

Many pts with a discoid lateral meniscus complain of knee popping or clunking, especially at extremes of motion.

- Other common complaints include a "bulge" at the lateral knee, pain, swelling, or locking.
- Many lateral meniscal variants (LMVs) are asymptomatic and found incidentally.

Did the pt sustain an injury?
Symptomatic LMVs have an insidious onset; a history of trauma resulting in knee pain is more likely due to a meniscal tear.

O   **Perform physical exam**
As these are often asymptomatic, the physical exam may be normal.
Findings may include:

- Bulge at the anterolateral knee with flexion

  ◆ Most commonly seen with unstable variants in children
- Range of motion may be limited by mechanical block.
  ◆ This can also be seen with meniscal tears.
- Flexed knee with ambulation
- Quadriceps atrophy (may be symmetric if bilateral discoid menisci)

Obtain x-rays of the knee
Anteroposterior, lateral, and Merchant views are adequate.
- Findings, if present, are usually subtle.

- The most common finding is a widened lateral joint space.

- Other findings include flattening of the lateral femoral condyle, lateral joint lipping, and lateral tibial plateau cupping.

Use MRI, arthrography, and/or arthroscopic evaluation to confirm the diagnosis

The classic finding on MRI continuity of the anterior and posterior horns on three or more contiguous 5-mm sagittal cuts (normally only seen in two).

- Nondiscoid variants of normal shape (but unstable) may appear normal.

A   **Lateral meniscal variant**
The prevalence of LMV is unknown due to the asymptomatic nature of many.
- The incidence has been reported to be as high as over 15% but is probably closer to 4%–5%.
The etiology of LMV is indeterminate; theories range from abnormalities of embryologic development to deformation from repeated trauma.
Variants can involve the entire meniscus or only part of it.
- Most common: discoid meniscus (greater thickness and tibial coverage)
- Other variants may include morphologically normal menisci that are hypermobile and "circular" menisci.
Anatomy
- While the medial meniscus is C shaped, the lateral meniscus is more circular and covers most of the lateral tibial plateau.
- The normal lateral meniscus is more mobile than the medial meniscus.
  ◆ This allows for greater excursion of the lateral femoral condyle, part of the "screw home" mechanism of terminal knee extension.
- The lateral meniscus is attached to the tibia anteriorly and posteriorly and often to the femur (through the meniscofemoral ligaments of Humphrey and Wrisberg).
- The average height of the normal lateral meniscus is 4–5 mm.

Classification of discoid lateral menisci
- Incomplete, complete, or Wrisberg's variant
  - Complete discoid lateral menisci essentially cover the lateral plateau whereas incomplete demonstrate increased size.
  - Wrsiberg's variant can either be normal or discoid morphology, but the essential feature is lack of a posterior tibial attachment resulting in hypermobility.

Symptoms are related to stability (hypermobility) of the lateral meniscus

Observe asymptomatic variants

Removal of a painless lateral meniscus results in development of early arthritis.

Surgery for symptomatic lesions depends on morphology, tears, and mobility
Arthroscopy is used to visualize and excise the abnormal tissue.
- A posterior portal may be required to access the lateral compartment.
- For total meniscectomy, open procedures may be technically easier.

Treatment of stable symptomatic lesions
- Historical treatment was resection (total meniscectomy), and some surgeons still prefer this because they feel the abnormal tissue will remain abnormal in function.
- "Saucerization" is now used by some to create a more normal-shaped lateral meniscus.
  - This is also suggested in tears to attempt to preserve some meniscal tissue, especially in children.

Treatment of unstable symptomatic lesions
- Total excision is generally recommended for these lesions.
- However, the goal of maintaining some meniscus in children has prompted some surgeons to attempt repair and reattachment of these mobile lesions.

Outcomes after surgery are largely dictated by age
Degenerative changes, advanced age, and female gender are associated with worse outcomes.
- Open and arthroscopic procedures have similar success rates.
- Young children with total or subtotal meniscectomies almost always develop radiographic arthritis but usually remain clinically asymptomatic.

S   What caused the injury?

Most distal radius fractures are the result of falls on an outstretched hand.

Does the pt lead an active lifestyle?
A fracture in the dominant wrist of a young athlete warrants more aggressive treatment
than that of a 90-year-old nursing home pt because the functional demands on the
wrist are different.

Can the pt be compliant with a postoperative plan?
A pt's history of substance abuse or other social issues suggests that the simplest
treatment plan should be considered.

O   Examine the pt
Skin: is the skin intact or is significant swelling present?
- Open fractures are a surgical emergency.
- Severe swelling may warrant admission for ice and elevation.

Marked deformity of the wrist may be noted with tenderness to palpation.
Neuro: median, radial, and ulnar nerves should be assessed for both sensory and
motor function.

> - Most commonly affected nerve is median, which can be involved in an acute
>   carpal tunnel syndrome.
>   - The carpal tunnel must be emergently decompressed in the operating room.

Vascular: radial pulse, capillary refill, and finger color
- Vascular injuries are rare except in cases of very-high-energy or penetrating
  injuries.

Shoulder and elbow should be assessed for pain and range of motion.
- Concomitant injuries to these joints are not uncommon with falls.

Palpate the scaphoid and perform the load test.

> - Scaphoid fractures are also often seen with distal radius fractures and are often
>   not visible radiographically.

Obtain x-rays of the wrist
Anteroposterior and lateral views of the wrist are used.
- Location: intra-articular versus extra-articular
- Step-off and gapping of fragments (especially intra-articular)
- Angulation of fracture: dorsal or volar
- Radial length: distance between the tip of radial styloid and ulna (12–15 mm)
- Radial inclination: normally 23 degrees
- Palmar tilt: normally 11 degrees

Various classification schemes have been developed for distal radius fractures, but
the reproducibility and clinical value of any of them is unproven.
The carpal bones and forearm/elbow should also be evaluated with plain films to
rule out concomitant injury.

Use CT and/or fluoroscopy if needed
CT scans of the wrist offer a better three-dimensional image of the fracture, particularly
if intra-articular extension is present.
- Sometimes the scaphoid impacts the distal radius creating an unimpressive injury
  on x-ray, but significant damage to the joint surface can be seen on CT scan.

Fluoroscopic evaluation of the fracture under anesthesia can also be used to determine
the personality of the fracture, but it carries the risks of anesthesia.

Distal radius fracture

One of the most common fractures, accounting for almost 20% of all fractures.

- Seen more often with advancing age (also common in younger children)
- Women are affected more often than men.

Historical treatments were generally nonoperative due to belief that almost universal return to painless, normal function could be expected.

- It is now known that the functional demands of the pt as well as the personality of the fracture should be used to determine treatment.

 Use stability to determine treatment of extra-articular fractures

Closed reduction and placement in a short- or long-arm cast is usually effective for stable extra-articular fractures.

- X-rays should be reviewed every 1–2 wks to ensure that displacement has not occurred.
- Casts should also be changed at those times to account for the decreased swelling and atrophy from disuse.

If closed reduction is not effective or the reduction cannot be held, the fracture is considered unstable.

- Treatment options for unstable extra-articular distal radius fractures include percutaneous pinning, external fixation, and open reduction with internal fixation.

Range of motion of the fingers and elbow is begun immediately, and wrist exercises are initiated when radiographic evidence of healing is noted.

The goal in treatment of all fractures is restoration of anatomy

Even minimal change in the normal anatomy changes the biomechanics and function of the wrist significantly.

- More than 1–2 mm of articular surface incongruity results in degenerative changes.
- More than 20 degrees of dorsal angulation or less than 10 degrees of radial inclination results in loss of grip strength and endurance.
- Radial shortening of 2.5 mm more than doubles the load borne by the distal ulna, resulting in pain and limitations in motion.

Cast non-displaced and stable intra-articular fractures

Due to the nearly anatomic reduction needed for the articular surfaces, many more of these injuries are treated with open reduction and internal fixation.

- Postoperative plan is similar to that for extra-articular fractures.

S

What is the pt's primary complaint?
Pts with degenerative osteoarthritis of the knee typically complain of pain.
Other common complaints include instability and mechanical dysfunction.
- Knee catching, locking, or "giving out"

How does the pt describe the pain? Do certain activities make it worse?
Pain is usually worsened with activity and often with weather changes.
Rest pain may be noted with advanced arthritis.
Difficulty with activities is common.

Stair climbing, prolonged walking, and squatting are challenging.

Is there a recent or distant history of trauma?
Degenerative changes often develop years after bone or soft tissue injuries.
- It is important to know whether the symptoms may be due to an acute fracture or soft tissue (cartilage, ligament) injury.

Does the pt have any medical comorbidities?
Osteoarthritis often occurs in older individuals, many of whom have medical conditions that should be addressed and may alter treatment options.

O

Perform physical exam
Gait evaluation: is the gait painless, is any knee thrust present, is alignment normal?
- Often an antalgic (painful) gait is noted.
- Medial or lateral thrust of the knees suggests severe deformity or instability.
- Excessive varus or valgus alignment may be seen after meniscectomy or with longstanding primary or secondary osteoarthritis.

Effusions and joint line tenderness are seen with advanced degeneration and meniscal pathologic lesions.
- Steinmann's and McMurray's tests are used to assess the menisci.

Crepitus with flexion-extension is often found.
Joint laxity may be noted due to either stretching or injury to the supporting ligaments.
- The cruciate ligaments should also be evaluated for integrity.

Range of motion (ROM) is often limited, though less so in active individuals.
- Many pts will present with a flexion contracture of 5–10 degrees.

The patellofemoral joint should be examined for pain, tracking, and stability.

Always examine the back, hip, and contralateral knee!
- Degenerative joint disease of the hip may present with knee pain.

Obtain weight–bearing x-rays
Anteroposterior (AP), lateral, and sunrise views of the knee
- All three compartments are evaluated: medial, lateral, and patellofemoral.

  ◆ Findings include joint space narrowing, osteophytes, subchondral sclerosis, subchondral cysts, condylar flattening.

AP views from the hip to the ankle allow for evaluation of the anatomic axis and are useful for preoperative planning.

Obtain MRI if the diagnosis is in question
MRI is not required to make the diagnosis of osteoarthritis.
- If radiographs are equivocal, it allows for assessment of menisci, ligaments, and any osteochondral defects.

Osteoarthritis of the knee
Primary osteoarthritis is a progressive, degenerative process involving the articular cartilage and, later, bones of the knee.
- Prevalence increases after age 50 yrs.
- Up to 85% of individuals over age 65 have radiographic evidence of osteoarthritis.
- There is no association between activity levels and primary osteoarthritis.

Secondary osteoarthritis occurs at a younger age.
- Often posttraumatic (fracture)
- Meniscectomy markedly increases the likelihood of secondary osteoarthritis.

Conservative management should always be tried first
Lifestyle modifications: avoidance of high-impact activities, weight loss
Physical therapy: strengthening and ROM exercises
NSAIDs, especially COX 2 inhibitors
Steroid injections may help relieve symptoms.
- Should be limited to three or four injections per year

Glucosamine and chondroitin may slow progression.
Viscosupplementation involves injection of hyaluronate into the knee; early studies suggest that this may be highly efficacious in symptom relief.

Poor response to nonoperative modalities may necessitate surgery

Arthroscopic debridement has fallen out of favor
This was historically performed to remove loose bodies and attempt to restore joint symmetry.
- Recently, highly publicized studies have suggested no benefit.
- Still performed in many centers, though.

Younger pts often benefit from osteotomies
Varus deformities with medial compartment disease or valgus deformities in pts with lateral compartment disease often respond well to corrective osteotomy.
- Relief of symptoms is the result of "off-loading" the affected compartment.
- Older pts with disease in only one compartment may be treated with a unicompartmental arthroplasty.

Older pts and those with 2+ compartment involvement should receive total knee replacements
Avoidance of high-impact activities is essential to prolong the life of the implant.
- Swimming, walking, and biking are permitted without limits.

S **What are the pt's complaints?**

Usually, a small nodule in the palm that may be painless is the first symptom.

When these nodules do not cause discomfort, they are often ignored until significant motion is lost.

Often the nodule will have been present for many years and then seemingly suddenly start to grow.

What risk factors does the pt have?

Several risk factors have been identified:

- Positive family history (transmission is autosomal dominant)
  - Scandinavian (or a country conquered by the Vikings) ancestry
  - Social history (associated with EtOH abuse and smoking)
  - HIV
  - Trauma has been suggested, but never proven, to be a cause

O **Perform physical exam**

Small nodules near the distal palmar crease are seen initially.

- Nodules may or may not be tender to palpation.

Cords may be palpable extending toward and away from the nodule.

The palmar area is generally affected before the fingers.

- Ring and small fingers are usually the first fingers involved.

Nodules dominate in early disease.

- As the disease progresses, cords predominate and replace nodules.
- Cords may span outward toward several digits.
- By this point, fingers have marked flexion contractures.

Neurovascular exam is usually normal.

Knuckle pads (Garrod's nodes), penile involvement (Peyronie's disease), and plantar fibromatosis (Lederhose's disease) should also be evaluated.

- These findings are seen in pts with "Dupuytren's diathesis," a particularly aggressive form of the disease that tends to affect multiple digits on both hands and be recalcitrant to surgery.
- Garrod's nodes and Peyronie's and Lederhose's rarely require surgery.

Consider differential diagnosis

Several conditions present similarly to Dupuytren's.

- Trigger finger
- Contracture of finger flexor tendons
- Tumor
  - The location of the mass and the typical skin pitting suggest Dupuytren's.
  - Bilateral location of changes help confirm the diagnosis.

No lab studies or imaging are required

If any question exists as to whether the mass is a tumor, x-rays and MRI scan should be obtained and a biopsy performed.

Dupuytren's Contracture
Usually affects men over 40 years old with the aforementioned risk factors.
Ultimate cause seems to be localized ischemia leading to fibrosis of palmar tissue.
Fibroblastic proliferation results in strangulation of microvasculature, and thus more ischemia and then more fibroblasts.
Risk factors described above all lead to oxygen free radical production, which stimulates fibroblasts to grow.
Two major histologic cell types involved are the fibroblast and myofibroblast.

- Historically, it was felt that myofibroblast was the hallmark cell of Dupuytren's, but recent studies indicate that these cells are found in other parts of the body.

Fibroblasts tend to line areas of mechanical stress where there is local ischemia (cords).
Nodules consist of the myofibroblasts and function as contractile elements.

Review the palmar anatomy in an orthopedic anatomy book
Knowledge of the normal anatomy is essential for understanding the pathologic process.

 Consider nonoperative treatments
Historically, physical therapy, steroid injections, splints, and various topical agents have been used with no statistically validated success.

Recent studies with proteolytic enzymes injected into the hand to dissolve the cords show promise.

Plan surgery when certain indications are met
Metacarpophalangeal joint contractures of 40 degrees or greater in one finger.

- Other affected digits on that hand should also be addressed at that time.
- The "table top" test is considered positive when a pt cannot put the palm of the hand flat on the table and is indicative of a severe contracture.

Proximal interphalangeal contractures are debatable, with some surgeons advocating contracture release whenever the joint is involved and others waiting until the contracture is greater than 30 degrees.

Essentially, the goal of surgery is release and resection of the diseased tissue.

- Many different approaches and procedures exist, and an understanding of these necessitates thorough knowledge of palmar anatomy.
- Prevention of skin flap necrosis and healing complications necessitates detailed preoperative planning as these can be devastating.

Recurrence rates are higher in young pts with advanced disease.

Emphasize the importance of postoperative therapy
Several days after surgery, a volar-based splint is applied to the forearm with the fingers in full extension.
Passive range of motion (ROM), scar massage, and wound care are started immediately.
Begin active ROM immediately and strength exercises at 4 wks.
Night splinting is continued for 6 months.

How did the injury occur?
Elbow dislocations in adults are usually the result of a fall on an extended arm.

Has the elbow dislocated before?
Most elbow dislocations are stable after a brief period of immobilization following closed reduction.
- Those that dislocate recurrently tend to be associated with high-energy trauma (such as motor vehicle accident) and resultant fractures.

Examine the elbow
Skin: significant swelling is often noted.
- If a wound is present near the elbow, ensure that the joint capsule is not compromised by injecting normal saline into the joint.
  - Landmarks may be difficult to identify for saline load test but needle should be placed between radial head, olecranon, and lateral epicondyle.

Gross deformity of the elbow may be obvious.
Neurologic assessment: median, radial, and ulnar nerve function should be evaluated for both motor and sensation.
- Self-limited stretch injuries to the median and ulnar nerves are common.

Vascular injury is suggested by cyanosis, asymmetric pulses, or an expanding hematoma.
- Most injuries to the brachial artery involve stretching that causes a transient spasm.
  - Any question of arterial compromise warrants Doppler studies and arterial angiography.

Shoulder and wrist range of motion (ROM) and areas of tenderness should be noted.

Obtain x-rays of the elbow
Two or three views of the elbow are needed prior to any manipulation.
- Clinically, it may be impossible to determine whether deformity at the elbow is due to a dislocation or distal humerus fracture.

Any associated fractures should be noted prior to reduction.
- The "terrible triad" is a devastating injury to the elbow consisting of dislocation, radial head fracture, and coronoid fracture.

Elbow dislocation
Account for one fifth of dislocations (only the shoulder and fingers are dislocated more often)
Most often occur in younger, active individuals
Associated fractures and avulsions are common
- In younger individuals, avulsion of the epicondyles is seen.
- Older individuals are more likely to have radial head or neck fractures, coronoid avulsions, and capitellar fractures.
- Associated fractures are related to worse functional outcomes than are simple dislocations.

Classify the dislocation
Classification guides the reduction maneuver.
- Posterior/posterolateral: accounts for 80% of elbow dislocations.
- Medial, lateral, anterior, and divergent dislocations also occur.
  - These tend to be the result of high-energy injuries such as seen in industrial accidents.
  - Neurovascular compromise is common with these injuries.

P

Reduce the dislocation

After thorough neurovascular and radiographic assessment, the dislocated elbow should be reduced as soon as possible.

For posterior dislocations, the method is:

- Gentle forearm traction with countertraction on the arm
- Manipulation of any medial or lateral displacement
- Flexion of the arm
  - An appreciable clunk should be felt.
- The arm should then be placed in a splint in neutral rotation and 90 degrees of flexion.

Reduction of the less common dislocations involves similar principles but usually prolonged traction.

Confirm adequacy of the reduction

This is done with both x-rays showing a concentric reduction and by physical exam.

- The arm should be fully flexed and extended to determine the presence of any instability.
- Valgus and varus stress should be applied to the extended and flexed arm to evaluate for collateral ligament damage.

Initiate ROM exercises quickly with stable reductions

Immobilization should be discontinued after 1 wk if the reduction is stable and elbow exercises begun at that time.

- If reduction unstable, up to 3 wks of immobilization may be utilized.
  - >3 wks of immobilization results in elbow stiffness.

Address fractures associated with dislocations

Avulsion fractures of the epicondyles can be managed expectantly if concentric reduction of the elbow can be achieved.

- Radial head fractures associated with elbow dislocations have a far worse prognosis than simple radial head fractures.
- Olecranon fractures are associated with high-energy anterior dislocations and significant loss of motion.
- "Terrible triad" injuries should be addressed semi-emergently to decrease the likelihood of heterotopic ossification and loss of elbow motion.

S **How did the injury occur?**
Different mechanisms are common causes for older and younger pts.
- Elderly pts frequently have a low-energy injury, such as a slip and fall.
- Younger pts typically sustain the injury as the result of a fall from significant height or motor vehicle accident (MVA).

If the pt had a slip and fall, investigate the reason.
- Was there an episode of light-headedness or syncope?

How does the pt describe the pain?
Chief complaint is usually severe hip pain with inability to bear weight.
- Younger pts often have associated injuries; thus their chief complaint may be unrelated to the hip injury.

Obtain past medical and social history
Concomitant medical problems and medications may predispose elderly pts to falling.
- Neurologically impaired pts are at an especially increased risk of falls.

Younger pts are often involved in drug and alcohol use when the injury occurs.

O **Perform physical exam**
General: vital signs and mental status should be assessed.
- In younger pts, the energy of the injury predisposes to life-threatening injuries.
- In older pts, the fall may be the result of an exacerbated medical problem.

Hip and leg: sensation, active and passive range of motion, vascular status
- Leg may appear normal or shortened and rotated.
- With low-energy mechanisms, neurovascular injuries are uncommon.
- In high-energy falls and MVAs, associated fractures in the ipsilateral leg are not uncommon and there is an increased likelihood of neurovascular dysfunction.

Full-body physical exam should be performed when other injuries are suspected or when the pt's general medical condition is compromised.

Evaluate x-rays
Anteroposterior (AP) pelvis and AP and lateral hip and femur should be obtained.
- If any other fractures are noted, films through the joints above and below the injured bone should be viewed.

MRI can also be utilized to detect an occult fracture if none is seen on x-ray.

Preoperative labs should be sent
In young, healthy trauma pts, CBC, ABG, and coags are sufficient.
Older pts require a more extensive workup, including any studies germane to their underlying medical issues.

Femoral neck fracture

Incidence of femoral neck and intertrochanteric fractures is about equal.
- Almost 3:1 male-to-female ratio
- Higher energy fractures and those with greater displacement/comminution are associated with higher nonunion and osteonecrosis rates.
- Delays in diagnosis and management are also associated with higher complication rates.
- Osteonecrosis develops from disruption of the lateral epiphysial artery (the terminal branch of the medial femoral circumflex), which is the main blood supply to the head.

Two classification schemes are of value
Garden's: based on radiographic displacement; useful for planning operative intervention.
- I—incomplete, non-displaced, valgus-impacted fracture
- II—complete non-displaced fracture
- III—partial displacement
- IV—complete displacement

Pauwel's: based on orientation of fracture line; an increased risk of osteonecrosis of the femoral head and nonunion of the neck is noted with a more vertical orientation.

Management is surgical
The treatment is dictated by the fracture pattern and the age and health of the pt. Non-displaced fractures (Garden I and II) should be fixed in situ with three or four pins or screws in a parallel orientation.
- Nonunion occurs in less than 5% of non-displaced fractures, and osteonecrosis occurs in less than 10%.
- This has historically been considered a surgical emergency in younger pts (younger than 40–50 years).
- Some authors have suggested that Garden I fractures (which are inherently stable) can be managed nonoperatively with toe touch weight bearing.
  - A displacement rate of up to 15% has been noted with this management.

Management of displaced fractures differs by age
In older pts, displaced (Garden III and IV) fractures are best managed with a cemented hemiarthroplasty.
- Hemiarthroplasty is also indicated in pts with metabolic bone disease.
- Debates with regards to hemiarthroplasty include approach (anterior versus posterior) and unipolar versus bipolar constructs.
- Total hip arthroplasty should be performed in pts with pre-existing hip disease.

Younger, active pts present a challenge as emergent reduction and pinning is recommended by most authors.
- The adequacy of the reduction is the most important factor in achieving union.
- Prompt reduction, though advocated by nearly all authors, has not been proven to reduce rates of nonunion or osteonecrosis (up to 30% and 33%, respectively).
- If closed reduction cannot be obtained, open reduction with screw and side plate fixation is appropriate.

Mortality rate in elderly pts approaches 30%
This is from all causes and is associated with the concomitant medical conditions as well as surgical complications.

S

How did the injury occur?
Forearm fractures in adults are usually the result of a high-energy impact such as motor vehicle accident.
- Lower energy injuries are seen with direct blows to the arm.

Does the pt have any medical conditions that preclude surgical management?
Most diaphyseal forearm fractures in adults are best managed with open reduction and internal fixation.
- Cardiac or hematologic abnormalities, for example, should be urgently addressed to allow for operative fixation of the fracture.

O

Examine the forearm, elbow, and wrist
Skin: significant swelling and integrity of the soft tissue must be assessed.
Range of motion (ROM): pain or limitation of ROM at the elbow or wrist suggests concomitant injury.
Deformity may be seen at the forearm, wrist, or elbow.
Neurologic function: assessment of sensory and motor function

- Injuries to nerves are rare, though the posterior interosseous nerve has been associated with Monteggia's fractures.

- Most of these injuries are self-limiting neurapraxias except in cases of mangling injuries.
Vascular status of the hand should be compared with that of contralateral side.
- Vascular injuries are also uncommon and usually involve the laceration of a single artery that does not endanger the hand (and thus needs no repair).
Monitor for signs of compartment syndrome: especially important with high-energy injuries; in intubated pts, the only sign will be tight compartments.

Obtain x-rays to evaluate the elbow through the wrist
Three views of the elbow, two of the forearm, and two or three of the wrist are essential.
- Many combined injuries are seen with forearm fractures, and proper management begins with knowledge of the full extent of the injury.

A

Forearm fracture
Range from low-energy nightstick injuries to severely comminuted fractures.
Generally, nonoperative treatments have fared terribly with regard to union and function.
The forearm is similar to a joint in that supination and pronation are functions of forearm rotation.
- For that reason, reduction must be as anatomic as possible to ensure that there is no forearm "joint" incongruity.

Classify the injury based on the physical exam and x-rays
Isolated ulna shaft fracture: usually caused by a direct blow to the forearm; this is also called the "nightstick fracture".
Isolated radial shaft fracture: can also be caused by a direct blow or fall.

- Isolated radial shaft fractures should raise the suspicion of an injury to the distal radial-ulna joint (Galeazzi's fracture).
Monteggia's fracture: Ulna fracture with dislocation of the radial head

- Type I: Ulna shaft fracture with anterior dislocation of radial head
- Type II: Ulna shaft fracture with posterior dislocation of radial head
- Type III: Ulna metaphysis fracture with lateral or anterolateral dislocation of radial head
- Type IV: Proximal both bone forearm fracture with anterior dislocation of the radial head
Both bone forearm fracture: usually a high-energy impaction or load injury

P   Isolated ulna shaft fracture

When displacement of the fracture is less than 50% of the diameter of the shaft and angulation less than 10 degrees, these injuries can be treated nonoperatively.
- The use of an ulna fracture brace allows immediate return to function as tolerated.
- If angulation or displacement is significant, an injury at the wrist must be suspected and open reduction, internal fixation is indicated.

Radial shaft fracture
Open reduction with internal fixation is almost universally warranted (unless the fracture is completely non-displaced).
- A non-displaced fracture may be managed with long-arm cast immobilization.
- Maintenance of anatomic alignment and radius length is essential to prevent loss of pronation/supination as well as disproportionate force distribution to the distal ulna
- If the distal radioulnar joint is involved, it should be reduced and pinned in full supination

Monteggia's fracture
The dislocation should be immediately reduced closed in the emergency room, if possible
- If this is not possible, the pt should be emergently taken to the operating room
- The ulna should be rigidly fixed with compression plating
- This will often allow closed radial head reduction
- If not, the radial head must be exposed and the interposed soft tissue extracted
Postoperatively, the arm should be immobilized for 4–6 wks

Both bone forearm fracture
Open reduction and internal fixation of both bones with compression plating
- Early return to ROM at the wrist and elbow improves function

Rigid fixation of diaphyseal injuries allows for return to activities of living
Avoidance of impact and heavy lifting for 3–4 months is the main limitation for nearly all forearm fractures managed with internal fixation

S

What are the chief complaints?

Pts with a pyogenic flexor tendon synovitis complain of severe pain on the volar aspect of their finger and pain with movement of the digit.

- Sometimes fever and general malaise

Was there any recent trauma?

Was the finger crushed or has the pt sustained an injury that penetrated the skin? Does the pt engage in heavy manual labor during which a nonpenetrating injury may have ruptured a tendon? (Presents with pain and limited movement.)

Discuss the medical social histories

Pts with a history of IV drug use, diabetes, HIV, cancer, or any other immunocompromised state are at a higher risk of an infectious cause for their complaints.

Does the pt suffer from any conditions that may be associated with tendon ruptures?

- Rheumatoid arthritis, repeated steroid injections into tendons

Pts who smoke generally have a more difficult time in resolving infections, particularly of the extremities.

- Smoking limits distal blood flow by vasoconstriction and (in the long term) results in structural changes in the blood vessels.

O

Perform a physical exam

General: look for signs of systemic illness.

- Fever, increased heart rate, blood pressure disturbances

Skin: evaluate for other areas of erythema, swelling, induration.

Hand: look for Kanavel's signs.

- Four cardinal signs of Kanavel suggest a diagnosis of suppurative flexor tendon synovitis:
  - ◆ Flexed posture of affected finger
  - ◆ Fusiform swelling
  - ◆ Tenderness over the flexor tendon sheath
  - ◆ Pain with passive extension of the finger

It is also important to note whether the infection has spread into the palm or adjacent fingers.

The sheath of the thumb is contiguous with the radial bursa and the sheath of the small finger is contiguous with the ulnar bursa.

- These two bursae communicate in up to 80% of the population and lend themselves to the development of a "horseshoe abscess."

Strength and range of motion of the superficial and deep flexor tendons should be evaluated to ensure they are intact if the exam is not consistent with flexor tendon synovitis.

Obtain plain x-rays of the hand

Three views of the hand and fingers should be obtained.

- Evaluate for fracture, dislocation, presence of foreign body, periosteal reaction (suggestive of bone involvement or osteomyelitis).

The clinical exam is quite reliable, and other radiographic studies such as ultrasound, CT, and MRI are usually not necessary.

Send labs

CBC with differential (look for elevated WBC and left shift)

Metabolic profile (especially important if pt clinically ill)

Coags (preoperative evaluation)

Acute phase reactants ESR and CRP (allow for evaluation of response to treatment)

Cultures should be sent for Gram stain and speciation.

Flexor Tendon Synovitis

In the face of the clinical exam, a diagnosis of suppurative flexor tendon synovitis can be made.

Definition: a pyogenic infection of the flexor tendon sheath

Other common infections of the hand include:

- Felon: infection of the deep pulp of the fingertip
- Paronychia: infection of the eponychial nail fold
- Herpetic whitlow: common in children and health care workers, it is a self-limiting vesicular reaction caused by exposure to herpes-infected orotracheal secretions.
- Septic joints: pain is generally more localized to that specific joint.
- Cellulitis: superficial infection of the skin
- Abscess: deeper infection, usually of the subcutaneous tissue though deep space abscesses do occur in the hands.

Initial treatment can be nonoperative

Early flexor tendon synovitis can be managed with 24 hrs of IV antibiotics; if this is effective, surgery can be avoided. PO antibiotics should be continued 7–10 days.

- *Staphylococcus* is the most common infectious agent; *Streptococcus* and gram-negative organisms are also found, and atypical mycobacteria are rare.

Surgical intervention is often necessary

Limited incisions are popular, with a small incision made at the A1 pulley (distal palmar crease) and another at the distal interphalangeal joint to allow irrigation of the sheath.

In cases where gross purulence is noted, an open debridement exposing the full length of the sheath is required.

Postoperative plan

Aggressive occupational therapy, IV (later PO) antibiotics, TID soap and water washes. Reoperation is usually unnecessary but should be performed if symptoms warrant.

S

What are the pt's complaints?
Complaints with hallux valgus can include cosmesis, shoe fit, transfer metatarsalgia, and deformity of the second toe.

What is the pt's profession?
Pts with high-demand professions or lifestyles must carefully weigh the risks and benefits of foot surgery (professional athletes, for example).

What does the pt expect from the surgery?
Improvement in cosmesis is a weak indication to perform the surgery.

- Improvement in shoe fit and pain reduction are more acceptable.

Obtain past medical history
Persons with diabetes, vasculopathy, or immunocompromise are generally poor surgical candidates for elective foot surgery.
- Complications, including infection and amputation, are common.

O

Perform physical exam
Evaluate pt in standing position.
- Observe arch of foot (normal, flat, or cavus), alignment of lower extremities, and position of great toe.

Foot and ankle, not just first toe, are fully examined
Neurovascular status of the foot should be assessed first (otherwise it may be skipped).
Range of motion (ROM) of ankle and subtalar joints to assess stability
Achilles tendon tightness (especially in juveniles)

ROM of great toe and the ability of the toe to be placed in neutral
- These are key indicators of how much correction is possible surgically.

Sesamoids should be evaluated for tenderness.
- Sesamoiditis may be the cause of the foot pain.
Osteophytes (dorsal) may cause pain and limit ROM.
Plantar callosities under the second metatarsal may indicate great toe instability.
Pain, crepitation, and stability of all Lisfranc and Chopart joints with ROM should be assessed.

Obtain radiographs
Three views of weight-bearing radiographs should always be obtained (anteroposterior, lateral, oblique).
If sesamoid pathologic process is suspected, then special sesamoid views are appropriate as well.
The following factors should be assessed radiographically:

- Hallux valgus angle: the angle between the long axes of the proximal phalanx and first metatarsal (normally <15 degrees); identifies metatarsophalangeal (MTP) joint deformity.
  - Intermetatarsal angle: the angle between the first and second metatarsals (normally less than 10 degrees); identifies metatarsus primus varus.
  - Hallux valgus interphalangeus: the angle between the long axes of the first proximal and distal phalanx (normally <10 degrees); identifies interphalangeal joint deformity.
  - Distal metatarsal articular angle: the angle between the shaft of the first metatarsal and a line through the base of the articular cap (normally <10 degrees); deformity predisposes to hallux valgus.

Other issues that should be looked at radiographically include the sesamoid positions, overall joint congruity, and any development of arthrosis.

Further imaging studies and labs are usually not needed
Pts with other medical problems who may be at increased risk of healing complications should have appropriate workups (blood flow studies in vascular pts).

Hallux valgus
The diagnosis is made on clinical grounds and evaluated radiographically to consider treatment options.
It is not a single deformity but a series of deformities that affect multiple joints in multiple toes. When the hallux valgus angle is increased:
- The abductor hallucis (a medial structure) is pulled laterally.
- The medial joint capsule remains as the only medially restraining structure.
- The adductor hallucis pulls the great toe farther laterally.
- The sesamoids are pulled medially, flattening the sesamoid ridge and worsening the deformity.
- The great toe rotates and pushes the lesser toes laterally.

Several factors are associated with the development of hallux valgus.
- Family history, pronated flat feet, posterior tibial tendon dysfunction, and joint incongruity of the first MTP joint

Consider nonoperative treatment initially
Wide-toe box shoes, insole padding, physical therapy, and activity modifications
- Extra-depth shoes are beneficial when concomitant lesser toe deformities are present (hammer toes, mallet toes).
- The bunion is often the primary location of pain; stretching the shoe leather over the bunion may also be helpful.

Surgery is indicated for pain that remains unimproved by conservative interventions
Before surgery is undertaken, it is essential to ensure that the pain is not the result of anything else (such as neuroma, wart, corns, and so forth).
A tremendous number of soft tissue and bony procedures have been described; discussion of these is well beyond the scope of this book.
- Considerations when choosing a procedure include the age of the pt (juveniles do poorly with isolated soft tissue procedures), degree of the deformity, congruity of the joint, and joint laxity.

S

How did the injury occur?
Usually the cause of the injury is clear.
- Falls, torsional injuries, penetrating trauma, motor vehicle crashes are common.

Is there pain anywhere else?
Especially important in higher energy trauma where associated injuries may occur

Does the pt have any other medical problems or previous injuries?
Previous fractures, metabolic or metastatic bone disease, neurologic injuries or disorders all impact the prognosis and treatment plan.

O

Perform physical exam
If the injury is the result of a polytrauma, the Advanced Trauma and Life Support guidelines should be followed ("ABCs") prior to evaluation of the extremity.
Skin: are there any abrasions or punctures that may suggest the fracture is open?
Motor and sensory exam: a thorough assessment of radial, median, and ulnar nerve function.
- Radial nerve palsies occur in up to 18% of humeral shaft fractures.
- Nine out of 10 resolve within 4 months.
- High association with distal third spiral fractures (Holstein–Lewis fracture)

Capillary refill and radial/ulnar pulses: evaluate for symmetry.
- Brachial artery injuries are rare but signify a surgical emergency.
- Asymmetry of pulses or hand color should raise suspicion and arteriography should be emergently performed.

Compartments should be monitored to ensure that compartment syndrome is not developing.
Ipsilateral shoulder and elbow should be evaluated for tenderness or pain with motion.

Obtain radiographs
Anteroposterior and lateral views of the humerus are required to evaluate the fracture.
- Location and pattern of the fracture dictate treatment options.
Views of the shoulder and elbow should also be reviewed.

Consider ultrasound if x-rays should be avoided
Pregnant women should avoid ionizing radiation if possible.

Work up pathologic fractures further
If the history or initial radiographic series suggests tumor or a metastatic process, CT, MRI, and bone scan may be required.
- Prior to fixation of a suspected pathologic fracture, the cause should be confirmed histologically.

Humeral shaft fracture
Relatively common injury in the U.S.
- Nearly 70,000 occur each year, accounting for 3% of all fractures.

Significant angulation and deformity can be accommodated due to mobility of shoulder and elbow joints; tolerance is tremendous.
- 20 degrees of angulation in the sagittal plane
- 30 degrees of angulation in the coronal plane
- 15 degrees of rotation
- 3 cm of shortening

P **Consider that most humeral shaft fractures can be managed nonoperatively**
Standard of care now involves the use of functional fracture bracing.
- Initially, a coaptation splint or hanging arm cast is applied (for 1 wk).
- The fracture brace is then applied as pain and swelling resolve.
- If tolerated by the pt, the fracture brace can be applied acutely.
- Slings may be used for up to 1 wk as well but should be discontinued after that time due to the likelihood of varus deformity developing.
- Once the brace is applied, activity is advanced as tolerated.
- The brace may be discontinued as soon as painless abduction of the arm is demonstrated.

Other nonoperative methods of immobilization are rarely used anymore
These include the shoulder spica cast and skeletal traction
- In elderly pts or children younger than 8 yrs, a sling and swathe may be used.

Consider indications for operative fixation
- Open fractures   - Multiple fractures
- Neurovascular compromise   - Segmental injuries
- Pathologic fractures   - Nonunion

Plan type of fixation
Compression plating of humeral shaft fractures is most commonly performed surgery.
Transverse, spiral, and segmental fractures treated surgically are best managed with the use of compression plates.
- Comminuted fractures may fare better with the use of a newer construct, the *locking plate.*
- Locking plates function as fixed-angle devices that allow moderate fracture motion and stimulate healing without further soft tissue damage.
External fixators may be indicated in open fractures in unstable pts.

Intramedullary nails tend to fail more often than plate fixation and are becoming less common.

S **How does the pt describe the pain?**
Pts will complain of pain in the hip and inability to bear weight.

Obtain history of event
Can be the result of direct or indirect forces
Twisting injury versus fall, though fall most common
Why did the injury occur?
- Did the pt suffer an episode of syncope as in a stroke or myocardial infarction (MI)?
- Has this happened before?
When did the injury occur?
- Older pts often fall at home and remain on the floor for 1–2 days.
- They often then present with dehydration, altered mental status, and renal problems.

Obtain detailed past medical history
Cardiovascular and neurologic disorders increase the likelihood of slips and falls and also should be addressed.
- It is also important to know about medications the pt is taking, such as anticoagulants.

Does the pt have risk factors for hip fractures?
Osteoporosis
Medical and psychological comorbidities (cardiac disease, unsteady gait)
Positive family history (a positive maternal history doubles the risk)

O **Perform physical exam**
General: vital signs and mental status should be quickly evaluated.
- Abnormalities should be immediately addressed.
Skin: integrity and quality of skin, bruising
- Excessive bruising suggests possible hematologic issues.
Lower extremity: often shortened and rotated
- Vascular injuries are rare but vascular status should be carefully assessed.
- Neurologic injuries are also uncommon.

Obtain x-rays
Anteroposterior (AP) of pelvis and AP and lateral plain films of the hip and femur should be evaluated.
Determination of stability is based on the plain film findings.
- Stability is primarily determined by the status of the posteromedial cortex of the proximal femur.
- Unstable fractures include those with posteromedial comminution, subtrochanteric extension, and fractures with a reverse obliquity pattern (fracture line extending from medial to lateral and distal).
- Stable fractures can resist compressive forces when reduced whereas unstable fractures displace or fall into varus.
Other radiographic assessment (CT, MRI) not necessary

Order preoperative studies
Usually managed by medical team; however, it is important to know what they will want:

- CBC	- Comprehensive metabolic profile
- PT, PTT, INR	- Chest x-ray
- ABG	- ECG

Intertrochanteric hip fracture
Diagnosed on radiographs though clinical history and physical exam are suggestive.
  • Accounts for almost half of proximal femur fractures in the U.S.
  • Incidence increases with age in both genders.
    • Female-male ratio is at least 2:1 (has been reported to be as high as 8:1).
    • Mortality rate from all causes is as high as 50% during the first year of injury.
It is imperative that any life-threatening comorbidity or condition be fully assessed
  by the appropriate consultant.

 Successful outcomes are only achieved with operative intervention
Stable and unstable fractures will both have poor outcomes if anatomic reduction
  with fixation is not done.
    • The primary goal is return to early ambulation; this improves functional
      outcomes and decreases mortality rates.
    • Surgery performed within 48 hrs of injury also decreases the mortality rate.
Partial or non–weight bearing on any extremity is difficult for the elderly.
    • Rigid constructs and anatomic reduction allow for early weight bearing as
      tolerated.

Various implants can be used for fixation

The most commonly used implant (and the gold standard) is the sliding hip com-
pression screw and side plate.
    • It maintains reduction while allowing micromovement and compression of
      the fracture fragments to stimulate healing.
    ♦ Cannot be used for reverse obliquity fractures.
Cephalomedullary nails have the benefit of percutaneous insertion.
    • The main problem with the use of these devices is failure at the tip of the nail,
      though design modifications have decreased the complication rate with this
      implant.
Other surgical options include the use of fixed-angle plates (best for reverse obliquity
  fracture patterns) and hemiarthroplasty.
    • Hemiarthroplasty is the most effective option for management of previous
      treatment failures.

Postoperative complications can be significant

Implant failure may occur in up to 15% of cases.
Infection which may become systemic or require further surgery.
Nonanatomic reductions resulting in malrotation or leg length discrepancy, rendering
  normal ambulation difficult.
Perioperative mortality: related both to the surgery (MI, pulmonary embolus) and to
  the underlying medical conditions that may have contributed to the injury in the
  first place.

S **Obtain history of the trauma**
These usually occur as the result of high-energy injuries.
- Motor vehicle accidents
- Falls from great heights

Lower energy injuries are associated with athletic participation.
- These are associated with a lower incidence of neurovascular injury.

What are the chief complaints?
Complaints include:
- Severe pain in the knee
- Inability to actively or passively move the knee
- Sometimes numbness or changes in sensation in the leg

Does the pt have any other areas of pain?
Knee dislocations are associated with fractures somewhere in the body in up to 60% of cases.
- This is due to the high-energy nature of most traumas associated with the injury and emphasizes the importance of a secondary survey.

 Perform physical exam
General: the entire pt must be evaluated.
- Assess vital signs (especially important due to likelihood of concomitant injury).
- Seemingly unaffected extremities and pelvis should be examined for pain and deformity.

Leg: focus the exam on the injured leg.
- Assess for deformity.
- Evaluate neurovascular status of leg distal to knee
  - Compare pulses with those of contralateral foot (KEY!).
  - Capillary refill and color should also be noted.
- Examine hip, thigh, leg, foot, and ankle for other areas of tenderness or deformity.
- Ensure that skin is intact.
  - Open dislocations require emergent surgery.

Obtain radiographs of the entire limb
Anteroposterior and lateral views of femur, knee, and tibia-fibula
- Most dislocations are anterior or posterior, although medial and lateral dislocations do occur.

CT and MRI are generally not acutely needed.
- CT may be obtained after reduction if a concomitant tibial plateau or distal femur fracture is noted.
- MRI is often needed to define extent of ligamentous injury.

Consider angiography
Angiography is usually not needed to assess popliteal artery.
Arterial competence can be safely monitored with Doppler studies.
- Abnormal pulses on Doppler, delayed capillary refill, or cyanosis warrant formal angiography.
- Pulse abnormalities can be due to spasm, but this is a diagnosis of exclusion.
- Failure to treat a popliteal artery injury within 8 hrs has been associated with an amputation rate as high as 85%.

Dislocated knee

Once the diagnosis is made, early management is essential.

Associated injuries must be evaluated.

- Ligamentous and capsular (anterior cruciate, posterior cruciate, lateral collateral, and medial collateral ligaments; joint capsule)
- Vascular injuries (popliteal artery injury in up to 40% of cases)
- Nerve injuries (usually neurapraxia involving common peroneal)
- Fractures (especially of tibial plateau)

 Reduce dislocation immediately

Can often be performed in emergency room without excessive sedation.

- If a dimple is noted medially, closed reduction should not be attempted because this indicates medial joint capsule interposition and is associated with an elevated risk of skin necrosis.
- If closed reduction is not possible, the emergent open reduction is needed.

Emergent surgery is sometimes necessary

Surgery cannot be delayed in certain situations.

- Irreducible dislocation
- Vascular injury
- Open dislocation
- Compartment syndrome

Definitive management

Essentially all surgeons recommend repair of any ligament ruptures subacutely.

- Nearly all dislocations are associated with compromise of at least one ligament.
- Exceptions include sedentary pts and those with stable knees after reduction.
- No consensus exists on how long after injury to repair the ligament injuries or the pre-repair management (immobilization versus range-of-motion exercises).
  - The minimum wait time appears to be 2 wks.

Nerve injuries are generally allowed 3 months for spontaneous improvement.

- Beyond that, nerve grafting is often required.
- A sharply transected nerve should be repaired acutely.

Outcomes are variable

Younger pts with fewer associated injuries (ligamentous, nervous, vascular) tend to fare better than older pts or those with multiple concomitant injuries.

S   Where is the pain?

Pain is noted at the lateral epicondyle, often with radiation into the forearm.

- It is usually exacerbated by activity.

Does the pt play tennis?

Repetitive ground strokes in tennis have been cited as the most common cause of lateral epicondylitis and are also responsible for the eponym.

What contributory recreational/occupational activities does the pt engage in?

Activities that may contribute include:

- Racquet sports   - Fencing
- Painting   - Raking

Is there any radiation of pain from the neck?

Cervical radiculopathy must always be considered when elbow pain, particularly with radiation, is present.

O   Examine the elbow

Tenderness to palpation will be noted over the lateral epicondyle.

- The origin of the extensor carpi radialis brevis is usually maximally tender.

Pain is exacerbated by resisted wrist and finger extension.

Range of motion is usually normal in the elbow and wrist.
Strength is usually normal.

- Weakness with resisted extension may be due to pain.

Sensation should be grossly intact.

- If sensation is abnormal, especially with associated weakness, cervical radiculopathy or radial nerve compression must be considered.

Obtain x-rays of the elbow

These are usually normal.
Anteroposterior and lateral views should be evaluated for completeness.

- Up to 25% of pts with lateral epicondylitis may have soft tissue calcification around the lateral epicondyle, but this is inconsequential.
- Plain films are also useful in evaluation of the elbow for degenerative changes or loose bodies.

If the diagnosis is clear, further workup is unnecessary

If the cause of the pain is unclear, further imaging studies of the elbow and neck may be required.

- Order electrodiagnostic studies of the radial nerve and posterior interosseous nerve if compression is suspected.

Lateral epicondylitis

Symptoms are caused by microtears within the substance of the extensor carpi radialis brevis endon.

Pathology may also involve other extensors (carpi longus or digitorum).

Up to 50% of tennis players will experience symptoms at some point.

- Usually occurs during fourth or fifth decade.
- Male and female rates are equal.
- Likelihood of developing symptoms directly related to time playing.
- Playing 2 or more hrs per wk increases risk up to 3.5-fold.

Development has been associated with several correctable risk factors.

- Poor stroke mechanics (leading into stroke with a flexed elbow)
- Improper racquet grip size, weight, and string tension
- Hard court play (ball moves faster and with greater momentum)

 Attempt conservative modalities

Pain control and relief of inflammation must be achieved first.

- Activity limitations without cessation of activity (avoid disuse complications)
- NSAIDs and ice

Consider corticosteroid injections into the deep tissue

Steroids should not be injected directly into the tendon (may precipitate rupture).

- Pain relief may initially occur in nearly 90% of pts.
- Long-term relief, however, is appreciated in probably less than half of pts.

Consider physical therapy with modalities

Physical therapy, ultrasound may be beneficial, but this has never been proven.

Once inflammation improves, modification of activities and equipment is begun

Return to sport with proper technique.

Use of lighter, loosely strung racquets with proper grip size.

Counterforce bracing: muscle firing is weaker, placing less stress on the injured tendon.

Further physical therapy focusing on strength, range of motion, and endurance.

6–12 months of nonoperative treatment may be required

Reported success rates range from 60% to 90% with prolonged treatment.

Consider surgery if conservative methods fail

Other causes of the pain must also be ruled out.

Procedure entails resection of pathologic tendon and reattachment to lateral epicondyle

- Up to 90% of pts have complete resolution of pain with surgery.
- Only 2% to 3% have no improvement.
- Main complications are weakness and pain.

S **What are the complaints?**
Children will usually complain of hip pain.

> • Knee pain is also commonly seen due to irritation of the obturator nerve, which extends down to the knee.

Parents will complain of a visible limp or altered gait.

Is the pain unilateral or bilateral?
Bilateral pain suggests another diagnosis, such as multiple epiphysial dysplasia.

Review risk factors
Family history
Low birth weight
Breech presentation at birth

Obtain medical and surgical history
Age of the child
  • Most commonly occurs in boys 4–8 yrs old
Was there a recent trauma?
  • Consider possibility of fracture or strain.
Has the child been ill recently?
  • Suggests possibility of transient synovitis.
Is the child currently ill?
  • Concern is septic hip, a true surgical emergency.
Does the child have a hormonal disorder?

> • Hypothyroidism and renal osteodystrophy are associated with slipped capital femoral epiphysis.

    ♦ A disorder of the proximal femoral physis seen in older, obese children

O **Perform physical exam**
General: evaluate for any general dysmorphic features that may suggest a genetic or chromosomal abnormality.
Hip: assess pain, range of motion (ROM), effusion.
  • Pain at the hip (and maybe knee) on active and passive ROM seen
  • Abduction and internal rotation are most limited.
  • An effusion is commonly present.
    ♦ Also seen with septic hip and transient synovitis.
  • The child may walk with an antalgic or Trendelenburg gait.
Knee: should also be evaluated if pain is present to rule out other cause of pain.

Obtain x-rays
Anteroposterior and frog-lateral views of the hip should be reviewed.
Degrees of osteonecrosis and head collapse are evaluated.
Other causes of hip pain (fractures, tumor) can also be seen.

Consider additional studies
In general, CT, MRI, and lab studies are not needed.
If the diagnosis is unclear or an underlying medical condition is suspected, then the appropriate studies should be performed.

Legg-Calvé-Perthes Disease (LCPD)
Diagnosis is made on clinical and radiographic grounds.
LCPD is a progressive, noninflammatory disorder of the proximal femur related to a vascular insult.
- Osteonecrosis of the proximal femoral epiphysis develops.
- LCPD progresses through four stages: initial, fragmentation, reossification, and healed.

Prognosis is dependent on both lateral pillar stage and bone age of the pt.
- Poor prognosis is conferred by bone age > 6 yrs, female gender, and decreased hip ROM (especially abduction).

Radiographic markers suggestive of poor prognosis include:
- Lateral subluxation   - Lateral calcification
- Metaphyseal cysts   - Horizontal growth plate
- Gage's sign (a lateral physeal defect)

The classification system now used is the Herring (or lateral pillar) classification
The lateral pillar of the capital femoral epiphysis is evaluated on the anteroposterior.
Divided into three groups with good predictability of prognosis.
- A: Little involvement of lateral pillar: good outcome
- B: >50% of height of lateral pillar maintained: good outcomes in younger pts (bone age <6 yrs) but poor outcomes in older children
- C: <50% of height of lateral pillar maintained: uniformly poor outcomes

Goals of treatment protocol are related to maintaining sphericity of femoral head
This is key in achieving a good functional result.
If the femoral head remains spherical:
- Pain is improved.
- ROM is maintained.
- Hip can be contained in anatomic position.

Control pain with NSAIDs and protected weight bearing
Weight bearing with crutches can be continued for several days to several weeks.

Restore ROM to achieve a good functional outcome
Consider inpatient or outpatient traction.
Selective muscle releases may diminish subluxing forces on the femoral head.
ROM exercises in a formal physical therapy program.
Casting can also be used.

The hip must be contained in the acetabulum
The treatments described for ROM are also useful in containing the femoral head in the acetabulum.
- Bracing the leg in abduction can also be utilized.
- If other treatments fail, pelvic or femoral (or both) osteotomy can be used to restore joint congruity and containment.

S **Obtain history of the trauma**

What was the mechanism of injury?
Injuries to the Lisfranc joint can be direct or indirect.

- Most are indirect, resulting from a combination of longitudinal and rotational forces (twisted foot striking the ground, for example).
- Direct injuries are caused by a crushing force applied directly to the joint as in a motor vehicle collision or fall from substantial height.
- Higher energy injuries (usually direct) are often associated with other injuries to the foot or body.

Where is the pain in the foot?
Midfoot pain after a fall or crush injury suggests Lisfranc joint injury.

Was the pt able to walk after the injury?
Ambulation is typically difficult following a Lisfranc injury.

Is there pain anywhere else?
Falls from heights or high-speed crashes should elicit concern over associated injuries.

O **Perform physical exam**
General: vital signs should be monitored, particularly in high-energy injuries where associated trauma is possible.
Foot: Pain, swelling, range of motion, compartment tension are all evaluated.

- Tenderness over the tarsometatarsal or midfoot pain with single heel rise is suggestive of a Lisfranc injury.
- Marked swelling of the skin with discoloration may be notable.
  - ◆ Ensure the skin is intact and the fracture is not open (surgical emergency).
- Range of motion and ability to bear weight are diminished.
- Compartment pressures should be evaluated clinically and measured objectively if they seem excessively tight or signs of compartment syndrome develop.

Ankle, leg, hip: should be evaluated on ipsilateral side to rule out concomitant injury.

Evaluate x-rays of the foot
Radiographic evaluation of the foot allows for assessment of stability of joint and associated injuries.
Views should be weight bearing if possible and include anteroposterior, lateral, and oblique.

- Disturbance in the relationship between the metatarsal bases and the tarsal bones on any view is indicative of a Lisfranc joint injury.
- The position of the second metatarsal relative to the middle cuneiform and the position of the fourth metatarsal relative to the base of the cuboid are the most sensitive predictors of injury to the joint.
- A "fleck sign" may be visible. This is an avulsion off either the medial cuneiform or the second metatarsal also indicative of injury.
- If the diagnosis is still in question, stress views may be beneficial.
- Views of the ankle should also be evaluated.

Classification is based on radiographs
Multiple schemes have been developed for the classification of these injuries and all take direction of displacement into account.

- None seem to be of value with regard to determining management or prognosis.

CT and MRI are usually not necessary
They can be helpful in preoperative planning and determining displacement.

Lisfranc joint injury
The Lisfranc joint proper is the tarsometatarsal joint.
The Lisfranc joint is part of the tarsometatarsal joint complex.
- This includes the metatarsals and cuneiforms, as well as the cuboid, navicular, and tarsometatarsal joints.

Injuries range from low-energy missteps to high-energy crushes with varying degrees of displacement and associated injuries.
Early diagnosis is essential.
- Even unimpressive radiographs may be associated with significant ligamentous injury.
- This often progresses to severe pain, instability, and arthritis.
- The diagnosis is initially missed in up to 20% of cases.
- Delays in diagnosis are associated with worse outcomes.

Determine treatment based one severity of injury and associated injuries

Displacement of less than 2 mm of the Lisfranc joint with no instability on stress views can be managed nonoperatively.
- These injuries should be treated with a short leg, non–weight-bearing cast for a minimum of 6 wks with radiographs after 1–2 wks to assess for further displacement.
- The same management is appropriate for those pts with midfoot tenderness or pain in the midfoot with ambulation (likely Lisfranc sprains).
- Following 6 wks of the non–weight-bearing cast, a walking cast should be used for 4–6 wks.
- Slow return to activities as tolerated follows.

Operatively fix displaced fractures
Instability or dislocation of the Lisfranc joint requires acquisition of anatomic reduction.
- This can usually be achieved with gentle axial traction.

Cannulated screws can be inserted under fluoroscopic guidance to maintain reduction.
Sometimes, wire fixation with 0.062 K-wires is adequate.
- If reduction cannot be achieved or maintained with percutaneous fixation, open reduction with internal fixation is necessary.

Be aware that results and complications vary
Closed reduction and casting of displaced fracture-dislocations has a much higher association with recurrent instability and posttraumatic arthritis than operative fixation.
The most debilitating complication of the acute injury is a missed compartment syndrome (CS).
- CS and open fractures are true surgical emergencies and are addressed immediately.

S   **What are the pt's complaints?**
Usually pain, weakness, and paresthesias

- Back pain is present in 95% of cases; leg pain in 71% (can be unilateral or bilateral).
- Exacerbated by prolonged standing and ambulation
- Improved by sitting or forward flexion of spine
- Pain and/or numbness is in lower extremities, usually in buttock region.
- Will also often complain of weakness or legs giving out

Nine out of 10 pts will complain of neurogenic claudication.

- This is a constellation of symptoms including leg pain, tightness, and weakness.
- Leaning forward as in pushing a grocery cart relieves the symptoms.

Gait disturbances, including tripping and instability, are common.
Bladder and bowel dysfunctions are uncommon but does occur.

- This is found in 10% to 15% of cases.

What risk factors for lumbar stenosis does the pt have?

- Previous trauma
- Previous spine surgery
- Achondroplasia
- Known spondylolisthesis
- Paget's disease
- Fluorosis

Obtain detailed medical history
This is important for considering differential diagnosis as well as treatment options.

Consider differential diagnosis
This is very broad and most easily done if broken down into systems.

- Vascular (acute aortic aneurysm, peripheral vascular disease)
- Musculoskeletal (degenerative joint disease, tumor)
- Neurologic (neuropathy, myelopathy)
- Miscellaneous (genitourinary, psychiatric)

O   **Perform physical exam**
Often, limited findings are noted on physical exam, even with severe symptoms.

- Tenderness to palpation may be noted in lumbosacral region.
- Muscle strength is usually normal in the lower extremities.
- If weakness is present, it is usually in the L5 root distribution.
- Weakness after exercise suggests the diagnosis of lumbar stenosis.
- Sensory exam will reveal decreased sensation in about 50% of pts.
- Deep tendon reflexes may be decreased, but this occurs commonly in the elderly.

Obtain plain x-rays to rule out pathologic conditions
These include tumors, fractures, and infections.

CT or MRI is needed to confirm and evaluate the diagnosis
Canals with a diameter less than 10 mm will show compression of the neural sac.

- MRI is especially helpful in evaluating all causes of sac compression, including hypertrophied ligamentum flavum or bulging disks.
- Electrophysiologic studies are generally not useful unless the diagnosis is not confirmed and peripheral neuropathy is suspected.

Degenerative lumbar stenosis (central)

Narrowing of the spinal canal, causing compression of the thecal sac (and thus nerve roots) and variable symptoms of pain, paresthesias, and weakness

- Disease is progressive and ultimately can become debilitating.
- Can be congenital (as in achondroplasia) or acquired (most common)
- Acquired stenosis is usually degenerative in origin.
- Symptoms typically develop in the fifth or sixth decade of life.
- Incidence ranges from 2% to 8% of the general population.
- No predilection exists based on gender, body habitus, or previous occupation.

Attempt conservative management initially

NSAIDs provide both pain relief and reduce inflammation.

- COX 2 inhibitors or enteric-coated aspirin have better gastrointestinal side effect profiles than traditional NSAIDs.

Weight loss, physical therapy, and core strengthening are often beneficial.

Oral corticosteroids can be utilized for pts with severe radicular symptoms.

- Complications include mental status and mood changes, endocrine disturbances, and the development of osteonecrosis of the proximal femur.

Braces can be used for short-term relief of pain.

- However, prolonged brace use has been associated with deconditioning of the truncal musculature and is no longer used.

Epidural steroid injections have shown variable results

Studies have shown anywhere from no clinical improvement to statistically significant improvement in the majority of cases.

- Epidural steroid injection is warranted as an attempt to avoid surgery or a definitive management in pts with significant medical comorbidities.
- However, complications can be severe and include paralysis, epidural hematoma formation, arachnoiditis, and meningitis.

Facet joint blocks have not been proven effective in lumbar stenosis

However, they are often helpful if the involved nerve roots can be definitively identified.

Operative decompression is effective (pain relief) in 80% to 85% of cases

Decompressions, with or without fusions, can be performed.

- Fusions are included in cases where either instability of flexion-extension films or listhesis is noted.
- Though outcomes tend to be favorable, complications can include infection, instability, hematoma formation, and failure of fusion.
- However, additional surgery is rarely required.

S

Where is the pain located?

In medial epicondylitis, discomfort is located along the medial elbow and worsened with activity.

Has the pt had a recent injury to the elbow?
Pain is usually insidious in onset.
- A recent trauma suggests that the pain is the result of an acute process such as a fracture or acute ligamentous injury.

What type of occupation is the pt involved in?
Persons involved in certain occupations are more likely to develop medial epicondylitis.
- Typists, bricklayers, and laborers who frequently use hammers

Does the pt engage in any recreational activities?
Golf, rowing, and throwing sports are associated with the development of medial epicondylitis.
- Golfer's elbow is actually more common in baseball players than golfers.

O

Perform physical exam
Tenderness to palpation is noted lateral and distal to the medial epicondyle.
- This area corresponds to the location of the flexor carpi radialis.
- Pain is worsened with resisted flexion and pronation of the forearm.
Range of motion of the elbow is usually normal.
Strength in the elbow and wrist is usually normal.
Sensation is generally intact.

Thoroughly evaluate elbow stability
Ligamentous instability must be considered whenever the diagnosis of medial epicondylitis is considered.
- Valgus stress testing with the forearm pronated will reveal laxity if the medial collateral ligaments are compromised.

Consider that a concomitant ulnar compression may exist
Changes in sensation in the small and ulnar ring finger suggest a possible compression of the ulnar nerve at the elbow.
- Pain and numbness will be noted in cases of ulnar nerve compression if the elbow is held flexed and the wrist extended for several minutes.

Obtain x-rays of the elbow
X-rays are usually normal.
Osteophytes and ligamentous calcification may be noted in pts with chronic overuse (pitchers).

CT and MRI are not necessary
If a ligamentous injury is suspected, MRI may be warranted.

Medial epicondylitis
Usually occurs during fourth to fifth decades
Male and female prevalence equal
Basically inflammation of the flexor-pronator mass of the arm
Mechanism of development is complex.

- Excessive valgus forces at the elbow stress the origin of the flexor-pronator group as well as the medial collateral ligament of the elbow
- Overuse, poor technique, poor conditioning, and inadequate warm-up can all lead to inflammation at the origin of the flexor-pronator mass.
- The flexor-pronator mass consists of the pronator teres, flexor carpi radialis, flexor carpi ulnaris, flexor digitorum superficialis, and palmaris longus.
    - The pronator teres and flexor carpi radialis are the most commonly affected muscles.
    - These muscles originate on the medial supracondylar ridge.
- One study showed that the flexor-pronator mass had visible tears in 100% of their pts who underwent surgery medial epicondylitis.

Attempt conservative treatment first

Medial epicondylitis generally responds to nonoperative treatment.

- Rest and avoidance of activity allow pain and inflammation to decrease.
- NSAIDs, ultrasound, and corticosteroid injections can also be used acutely.

Prevent the recurrence of inflammation once it is eradicated
Rehabilitation program is undertaken to improve strength, flexibility, endurance, and maintain range of motion.

- Modification of work-related and recreational activities with slow return to full activities follows.
- Counterforce braces are also sometimes helpful in the subacute phase.

Continue nonoperative interventions for a minimum of 6 months

Surgery should not be considered before this time since nonoperative treatment is usually effective.

Surgery focuses on releasing the damaged tissue from its origin
Historical operative techniques for medial epicondylitis cause significant weakness of the flexor-pronator.

- This weakness is debilitating for active laborers or athletes.
- However, pain is usually relieved.

Newer techniques focus on resection of the inflamed tissue and reapproximation of the healthy muscle
Return to normal activities is usually experienced by the fourth postoperative month.
In one study, all 20 athletes in whom the procedure was performed returned to sport.

Loss of strength after the procedure is still the major complication.

S

What are the chief complaints?
Catching, locking, and popping with pain of the knee are often noted.
- These can also be due to other abnormalities, such as degenerative joint disease or patellofemoral pathology.

Was there an acute injury?
Meniscal tears usually involve a twisting injury and are painful and swollen.
- Chronic meniscal tears are often atraumatic, or they may be the result of a forgotten trauma.
  - These pts will complain of chronic knee pain, mild to moderate swelling, and exacerbation of symptoms with activity.

O

Examine the pt
Observation: look at the knee.
- Look for effusion, atrophy of quadriceps, swelling along joint line (consistent with cyst formation).
Range of motion (ROM): assess active and passive.
- Often limited by pain and swelling acutely and pain chronically
  - Loss of full extension following an acute injury may suggest a displaced bucket handle tear, which requires urgent surgery (to maintain ROM).

Palpation
- Tenderness to palpation along the joint line is a hallmark and probably the most sensitive test.
- Also assess for patellofemoral, tendon, and collateral ligament tenderness.
- With a concomitant anterior cruciate ligament (ACL) injury, tenderness along the joint line is less reliable.
Special tests include the Steinmann, McMurray, and Apley tests.
- These have limited proven efficacy in diagnosis.
Assess ligamentous laxity of the ACL, posterior cruciate ligament, and collateral ligaments.

Obtain x-rays of the knees
Weight-bearing views of the knees with a 45-degree posteroanterior, standing true lateral, and Merchant view are useful for evaluating for the presence of fractures and degenerative changes.
- Meniscal tears cannot be seen on plain films.

If clinically suspicious, obtain an MRI
MRI has excellent sensitivity and specificity in diagnosing meniscal and other soft tissue injuries.
- Accuracy of newer MRI scans has been reported to be 95% for meniscal tears.
- Only images that are full thickness on MRI are truly tears (and not degeneration).

If the diagnosis is still in question, confirm with diagnostic arthroscopy
Direct visualization of the menisci is the most sensitive and accurate method of diagnosing meniscal tears.

Meniscal Tear

Meniscal tears can involve either the medial or lateral meniscus or both.

- They occur in about 60/100,000 per year and are more common in men > 40.
- About one third are associated with an injury to the ACL.
  - ◆ In these pts, lateral meniscal injuries are more common than medial whereas medial meniscal tears are otherwise more common.

Anatomy

The medial meniscus is a C-shaped piece of cartilage whereas the lateral is almost circular with a hollow center; both are affixed to the tibial plateau.

- They are also attached to each other, the femur, and the joint capsule of the knee through various ligaments.
- The main functions of the menisci are force distribution, shock absorption, maintenance of joint congruity, and increasing joint contact areas.

Menisci are relatively avascular structures.

- Only the peripheral 10% to 25% of the lateral and 10% to 30% of the medial meniscus has a blood supply, though in children under 10, more of the meniscus is vascular.

Determine whether this should be managed surgically

Most acute meniscal tears should be managed surgically; the question is whether to repair or resect.

Most meniscal surgery now is arthroscopic.

- Exceptions to surgery: partial-thickness tears, stable tears (cannot be moved with probe), small radial or longitudinal tears (less than 3 mm and 10 mm, respectively)
  - ◆ These tend to heal uneventfully.
- If possible, the menisci should be repaired with various suturing techniques.

  - ◆ Criteria for repair include tear size (>10 mm), location in the vascular (peripheral) zone, ligamentous stability (or concomitant repair), no degeneration of the tear, and an active pt

  - ◆ Repair in children whenever possible, even if not all criteria are met.
  - ◆ When ACL injury associated, repair should be attempted.
- If the menisci cannot be repaired, partial meniscectomy can be performed.
  - ◆ Goals are removal of loose fragments or unstable rims and smoothing of the rim (rim does not have to be perfect because it does remodel).

  - ◆ Err on the side of leaving too much menisci (can always cut more later but goal is to prevent degenerative arthritis).

- Some surgeons are now performing meniscal transplantations with allograft.
  - ◆ Results are variable and this procedure requires further evaluation.

Postoperative rehab is conservative; when ACL is also repaired, this dictates plan

Flexion and weight bearing are limited either way, though weight bearing after a concomitant ACL repair is usually with a knee brace locked in extension.

S **What are the chief complaints?**

Several complaints are common:

- In-toeing gait
- Cosmesis
- Excessive shoe wear

Does the child have any other medical problems?

Certain disorders, such as cerebral palsy, are associated with metatarsus adductus.

Is there a family history of other "packaging" abnormalities?

Internal tibial torsion and clubfoot are related to a tight intrauterine space.

Was there anything unusual in the birth history?

Complications of pregnancy and birth should be discussed.

Review risk factors

Several risk factors have been established:

- Males
- Twin births
- Preterm babies

O **Perform physical exam**

A thorough exam of the foot is required.

- Foot appears C shaped (concave medially and convex laterally).
- Toes point inward with gait (if able to walk).
- Skin is grossly normal.
- Hindfoot can be either in neutral or varus.
- Range of motion and strength of ankle and subtalar joint are normal.

Examine the entire pt to look for other abnormalities.

Obtain radiographs only in older children

Routine radiographs are not necessary in infants.

If child is >4 yrs old then x-rays are appropriate.

Classifications based on radiographs have poor inter- and intraobserver reliability.

Consider other potential causes of in-toeing gait

Many other causes of in-toeing gait have been described:

- Metatarsus primus varus
- Skewfoot
- Positional calcaneovalgus (especially in neonates and infants)
- Internal tibial torsion
- Femoral torsion

Metatarsus Adductus
Diagnosis is made on clinical grounds.
Most common pediatric foot problem referred to orthopedists.
- Previously believed to be associated with developmental hip dysplasia but this is not supported by recent studies.
- Occurs in 1 in 5000 live births.
- Occurs in 1 of 20 siblings of persons with metatarsus adductus.
- Usually occurs on left side.
- Most commonly noted in first year of life.

Classify the deformity
Metatarsus adductus can be based on heel bisector angle (line passing through middle of heel should pass between second and third toes).
- Mild: line passes through third toe.
- Moderate: line passes between third and fourth toes.
- Severe: line passes lateral to fourth toe.

Classification based on flexibility may be more valuable with regard to prognosis.
- Flexible: forefoot can be abducted beyond heel-bisector line.
- Partially flexible: forefoot can be abducted to midline.
- Rigid: cannot be abducted to midline.

Remember that this is usually a self-limiting disorder

Several studies have shown total or nearly complete resolution with no intervention.
- This is probably adequate for flexible or partially flexible cases.
- Resolution of deformity is the norm.
- More importantly, foot is painless in adulthood.
- Complete resolution may take several years.

Cast rigid deformities
Either long or short leg casts may be used.
- Casts must be worn for 6–8 total wks.
- Casts should be changed every 1–2 wks.
- Long-term outcomes have shown very rare return of deformity.

Surgery is rarely required but should be performed if necessary
Usual reason is painful show wear
Many procedures have been described with variable complications.
- Abductor hallucis tendon lengthening with medial capsulotomies of naviculo-cuneiform and cuneiform–first metatarsal joints has recently been shown effective and safe.
- The most accepted and safe procedure: opening wedge osteotomy of medial cuneiform with closing wedge osteotomy of cuboid.
    - Avoids risk of shortening of first metatarsal seen with metatarsal base osteotomies.
    - Also associated with minimal skin and wound healing complications

S **What are the pt's complaints?**
Pts with metastatic bone disease usually complain of pain at the sites of the metastases.

- Often, metastases are the first manifestation of a previously undiagnosed primary tumor.

Constitutional complaints are common
- Fever   - Night sweats
- Weight loss   - Fatigue

Pts may also present with an acute fracture and acute pain with inability to use the limb.
Findings may be incidental on radiographs taken for other reasons.

Review medical, family, and social history
How old is the pt?

- Destructive bone lesions in pts older than 40 yrs are metastatic bone disease until proven otherwise.

Does the pt have a history of cancer?
- A known history of cancer, even in remission, suggests metastatic disease.
Is there a family history of cancer?
Does the pt have any conditions that may mimic cancer?
- Bone cysts, fibrous dysplasia, Paget's disease, other metabolic bone diseases
Does the pt drink alcohol and/or smoke?
- Many carcinomas are associated with cigarette smoking and/or excessive EtOH.

 A solitary bone lesion in a pt older than 40 warrants a thorough workup starting with plain x-rays of the affected limb in two planes
Radiographs of metastatic carcinoma (most metastases are carcinomas) demonstrate a destructive, lytic lesion though mixed or even blastic lesions are possible.

Obtain a technetium bone scan
Even with no known primary tumor, multiple lesions must be ruled out.

Consider further radiographic evaluation
Chest x-ray and CT to evaluate for lung cancer.
Abdominal CT to evaluate for renal cell cancer, lymphoma, and colon cancer.
If multiple myeloma is suspected, a skeletal survey should be obtained.

Send labs
CBC with differential
- Evaluate for leukemia, lymphoma, anemia.
ESR (general marker of inflammation)
Serum and urine protein electrophoresis (Bence Jones protein in urine suggests myeloma)
Comprehensive metabolic profile to evaluate for any electrolyte, renal, or hepatic abnormalities

Obtain biopsy
Biopsy results confirm the diagnosis.
- Biopsies of carcinomas reveal epithelial cells arranged in a glandular pattern within a fibrous stroma.

Perform full physical exam
The physical exam is usually nondiagnostic with metastatic bone disease.

Metastatic bone disease

The most common cause of skeletal destruction in older pts.

Most common locations of metastases are pelvis, vertebrae, ribs, and proximal limb girdles.

Pathogenesis: Batson's venous plexus drains the blood from the breast, lung, thyroid, kidney, and prostate.

- These are also the five most common tumors found to metastasize to bone.
- The plexus is a valveless system that has an intimate relationship with the vertebral column, pelvis, and proximal limb girdle.

Destruction of bone is not a direct function of the tumor cells.

- Released cytokines stimulate osteoclastic activity and destruction of bone.

Assess the nature and severity of the disease

The type of tumor, the extent of spread, and the pt's overall health must be considered and the pt must be aware of the extent of his or her condition.

Control pain and maintain function

Metastatic disease is often a terminal condition and care is palliative.

Medical management consists of traditional pain control (NSAIDs, narcotics) and attempts to control bone destruction (slow osteoclast activity).

Bisphosphonates are used to combat excessive osteoclast activity.

- Older bisphosphonates (such as etidronic acid) inhibit both osteoclast activity and formation of new bone.
- IV pamidronate is now the bisphosphonate most commonly used.

Perform internal fixation if warranted

Any acute fracture requires internal fixation.

Fixation is easier and associated with fewer complications if performed prior to a fracture.

Prophylactic internal fixation is appropriate when certain risk factors are present.

- More than 50% cortical destruction in the diaphysis
- Extensive subtrochanteric femur destruction
- Extensive destruction of metaphyseal bone
- Marked pain persisting after irradiation (suggests possible stress or insufficiency fracture)
- Clinical judgment

The method of fixation utilized is dictated by the location and extent of the lesion.

Arrange for a multidisciplinary approach to address the primary cancer

The orthopedist, oncologist, radiation oncologist, and primary care physician must all work together to best manage this complicated condition.

S

Obtain history of pain

When did the pain begin?

Was it related to a traumatic event or has it occurred before?

- Tarsal tunnel syndrome, fractures, synovitis, Freiberg's infraction can all give similar symptoms.

Where is the pain located in the foot?

- Pain from Morton's neuroma is classically in the third web space of the foot with palpation.
    - Pts will often complain of diffuse forefoot discomfort and paresthesias in the two toes surrounding the web space.

What makes the pain better or worse?

- Pain with Morton's neuroma is usually exacerbated by wearing tight shoes and walking.
- Relief is generally appreciated by removal of the shoes and massage of the affected area.

O

Observe the pt

What type of shoes is the pt wearing?

- Morton's neuromas are far more common in those who wear high-heeled shoes with a tight toe box.
    - This is part of the reason they are 8–9 times more common in women.

Examine the pt

Evaluate the gait: Does the pt have an antalgic gait or any other abnormality?

Assess neurovascular status.

- Sensory deficits are uncommon in Morton's neuromas.
    - They are important to document as they help confirm the diagnosis.
    - It is equally important to determine that there is no other neurovascular explanation for the symptoms (e.g., tarsal tunnel syndrome).

Assess areas of tenderness.

- The third web space accounts for 80% of Morton's neuromas; the second about 20%. Tenderness to palpation in these areas is a *sin quo non* for a Morton's neuroma.

Obtain objective studies starting with x-rays

Three views on x-ray are needed to evaluate the foot for osseous abnormalities.

- X-rays are usually normal.
    - Carefully assess for evidence of fractures, osteochondritis dissecans (Freiberg's infraction), tumor, or any other radiographic abnormalities.

Nerve conduction velocity testing, MRI, and CT are not needed unless the diagnosis is in question; usually the physical exam and history are classic.

Bone scans are excellent for assessing the presence of a stress fracture in cases where the exam is equivocal.

Morton's Neuroma

The diagnosis is made on the basis of the physical exam.

These do not represent true neuromas.

- There is not a random, haphazard collection of axons as seen in neuromas.

The etiology is likely degenerative and related to repetitive microtrauma.

- This is supported by the histology (significant collagen and hyaline deposition is found).

The neuroma is found just plantar to the intermetatarsal ligament and often has a bulbous morphology.

- However, most Morton's neuromas do not appear grossly abnormal.
- Anatomically, they are found at the most distal portion of the common digital nerve.
  - The nerve then bifurcates into the proper digital nerves (medial and lateral).

Attempt nonsurgical management initially

Nonoperative treatment should be initiated prior to any operative resection.

- Wearing shoes with a wide toe box, stiff sole, and sometimes a metatarsal pad.

Steroid injections have questionable efficacy but are also an acceptable nonsurgical option.

Consider surgery if nonsurgical management fails

The common digital nerve can be operatively resected.

- It should be divided a minimum of 3 cm proximal to its bifurcation.
  - This will ensure that the stump is not in a weight-bearing area of the foot (and likely to remain symptomatic).

Surgical resection relieves pain in 80% to 85% of patients; residual numbness in the nerve's dermatome can be expected.

If the initial surgery fails, reoperation is possible

Re-excision is effective in relieving pain only 65% to 75% of the time.

- Most of the successes in revision surgery occur in cases where the nerve was initially cut too distal.
  - This leaves several plantar nerve branches intact.

Postoperative course is usually uncomplicated

Pts can be sent home the day of the surgery.

- May be weight bearing as tolerated in a wooden shoe.

Sutures are removed after 3 wks.

Return to normal activities after 6 wks.

S **Obtain history of event**
Often a recent history of high-velocity trauma to the head or neck
- Motor vehicle accidents often result in neck flexion or extension.

> ◆ 80% of odontoid fractures are the result of flexion injuries whereas 20% are the result of a primarily extension force.

In elderly pts, falls are a common mechanism.
- As the pt falls forward, he or she strikes the head on some object, causing a hyperextension injury.

What are the complaints?
Complaints are variable.
- High neck and/or head pain
- Pain in head is usually occipital.
- Changes in sensation or weakness are disconcerting symptoms that sometimes occur.
- Pts who are obtunded may not be able to localize pain.

O **Perform physical exam**
General: Is the pt alert or is there any other pain?
- Regardless of whether other areas of pain are present or the pt is obtunded, a complete exam is essential.

Neck: Range of motion (ROM) usually decreased, muscle spasms may be noted.
- In non-displaced fractures, however, the initial physical exam may reveal no pain on tenderness.
- The complete cervical spine must be examined in pts with any C-spine fracture.

Spine: tenderness, limited ROM may be present.

> - Noncontiguous spine fracture occurs in up to 10% of cases.

Head: commonly other facial trauma is evident; determination of injuries to upper cervical roots or cranial nerves should be performed.
- The greater occipital nerve is the most commonly injured structure.

Extremities: Evaluation of sensory and motor function of all extremities

> - Neurologic injuries occur in up to 25% of odontoid fractures.

- These injuries can range from complete paralysis to mild sensory disturbances involving a single nerve root.

A rectal exam should always be performed.
- Determination of sensation, tone, and volutional control are an essential part of any spine exam.

Obtain plain x-rays of the neck
The initial film series includes anteroposterior, lateral, and open mouth views of the C-spine.
- In awake pts, flexion-extension views are obtained to assess for any associated ligamentous injuries if no displacement is noted.
- If the pt is obtunded, physician-assisted fluoroscopic evaluation is needed.
- Views of the thoracic and lumbar spine and sacrum are reviewed as well.

Obtain CT scans with sagittal and coronal reconstructions

> With non-displaced fractures, however, fracture lines that are parallel to the CT plane may be missed, even with reconstructions.

MRI may be useful in determining ligamentous injuries
Injuries to the transverse ligament can cause significant instability; nonetheless, there is no consensus regarding the routine use of MRI.

Odontoid fracture
Accounts for 7% to 14% of all cervical spine fractures.
Early literature suggested nonunion rates of nearly 90%.

Classification is based on fracture level
This has been found to be predictive of the rate of nonunion.
- Type I: Avulsion of tip of odontoid (rare); transverse ligament remains intact
- Type II: Fracture at junction of odontoid and body of axis (most common); transverse ligament is often injured
  - Also most unstable and highest risk of nonunion
- Type III: Fracture extends into body of axis; usually not associated with transverse ligament injury.

Overall union rates have improved considerably, though nonunion rate for type II fractures has recently been reported as 15% to 85%.
It has been hypothesized that nonunion in type II fractures is related to disruption of the vascular anastomosis, which supplies that area of the odontoid.
- Nonunion in type II fractures is also associated with smoking, more than 4 mm displacement, and excessive angulation.

Plan treatment based on fracture type
Type I: Generally stable and thus usually requires no fixation
- Rigid C-collar for 8–12 wks is usually adequate

Type II: Management remains controversial due to high rates of nonunion
- Non-displaced type II fractures may be managed with halo immobilization for 12–16 wks but must be monitored closely for displacement.
- Displaced fractures can be managed with either atlantoaxial arthrodesis or anterior screw fixation.
  - Both have reported union rates of >90%

Type III: Generally stable; often requires reduction with tongs or halo
- Halo immobilization for 12–16 wks is associated with 90% union rates.

Manage nonunions surgically

Currently, the gold standard for nonunion of odontoid fractures is posterior fusion.
- Anterior screw fixation may be effective, but long-term data are limited.

S **What complaints does the child or caregiver have?**

The child refuses to use the affected extremity.

Older children complain of pain.
Constitutional (malaise, anorexia) complaints are less common

Is there a recent history of injury?
Contusions or fractures present similarly and there is often a history of trauma.
Consider the possibility of abuse.

Obtain a detailed medical history
This includes recent illnesses, systemic conditions, and family history.

O **Examine the pt**
Assess vital signs.
  • Fever is often, but not always, present.
Swelling may be present.
  • Cellulitis overlying a swollen area may suggest an abscess
Older children will have point tenderness on palpation.

  • Usually, older children can bear weight.

Younger children also have point tenderness.
  • However, they often are not able to bear weight or use the extremity.
Neonates often have impressive swelling and extreme irritability on movement.
  • Severe pain with movement of a joint elicits concern for pyarthrosis.

Obtain x-rays of the affected extremity
Useful for evaluating for infection as well as fractures (rule out abuse).

  • Osteolytic changes take 10 days to 2 wks to develop.
    ◆ Soft tissue swelling can be seen as early as 2 days.
    ◆ Periosteal reaction (new bone formation) is often evident within 1 wk.

Obtain other imaging modalities if the diagnosis is in question

MRI with gadolinium is the most sensitive and specific test for osteomyelitis.

Technetium bone scans have a positive predictive value similar to that of MRI but do
  not provide multiplanar images.
Indium-111–labeled white blood cell scans can be used when the technetium scan is
  normal but there is a high clinical suspicion for osteomyelitis.

  • Indium scans have a poor sensitivity for spinal osteomyelitis.

Send infection labs
CBC: white count is elevated only 40% of the time.
ESR: elevated in over 90% of cases of acute hematogenous osteomyelitis.
CRP: elevated in almost 100% of pts.
  • ESR and CRP are impacted by trauma, systemic illnesses, and recent surgery.
Blood cultures, direct bone cultures, and sometimes joint aspirates

  • Direct cultures are positive up to 85% of the time while blood cultures are positive
    less than 60% of the time.

  • If a septic joint is suspected, a joint aspirate should be sent for immediate
    Gram stain, cell count, protein, and glucose (and culture).

Consider the broad differential diagnosis
Remember to keep an open mind as the exam is nonspecific.
- Trauma (fractures, contusions, overuse)
- Infection (septic joint)
- Immunologic (rheumatic fever, transient synovitis, reactive arthritis)
- Tumor (osteosarcoma, Ewing's sarcoma)
- Other rare systemic conditions

Acute hematogenous osteomyelitis
Bacterial infection in the bones, which in children usually involve the metaphyseal bone.
- Seeding from the blood during transient bacteremia most common, though acute osteomyelitis may occur through direct inoculation or contiguous spread.
- Children are particularly susceptible due to the sluggish blood flow through the metaphyseal bone, which is an ideal environment for bacterial growth
- Neonates have epiphyseal vessels that cross the physis and provide bacterial access to joints where the metaphysis is intracapsular.
    - Shoulder, elbow, hip, and ankle are thus susceptible to concomitant septic arthritis when in the setting of acute osteomyelitis.

- *Staphylococcus aureus* accounts for 9 out of 10 cases.

    - Various streptococcal species account for most of the rest.
    - *Haemophilus influenzae* is rarely the cause in immunized children.

    - Group B *Streptococcus,* gram-negative rods are sometimes cultured in neonates.
    - Children with sickle cell have an increased incidence of *Salmonella* infection.

Management is usually nonoperative
Ideally, a species-specific parenteral antibiotic is selected, though empiric treatment is required while awaiting cultures or if they are negative
Coverage for *S. aureus* is always required because it is most common
- Antistaphylococcal penicillin with an aminoglycoside for neonates
- Cefuroxime can be a single agent given to children <3
- Cefazolin or antistaphylococcal penicillin for older children
- When cultures return a species, the coverage can be narrowed

Plan surgery if an abscess or necrotic bone is present
Debridement of a sequestrum or abscess is essential for eradicating the infection.
- Antibiotic penetration into abscesses and dead bone is ineffective.

Duration of IV antibiotic treatment is controversial; 5 days to 8 wks proposed
Usually, 1 wk of IV antibiotics followed by 3 wks of oral is effective; the ESR, CRP, and clinical appearance are the best indicators of infection eradication.

S

What are the presenting complaints?
Osteonecrosis can be clinically asymptomatic or associated with a variety of complaints. Pain is almost always present.
- Usually localized to groin but can involve buttock and knee.
- Onset is usually insidious.
- Quality is deep, intermittent, throbbing.

Review past medical and social history
How old is the pt?
- Average age of presentation is 38 years old.

Numerous causes of osteonecrosis have been described.

- Trauma	- Corticosteroid use
- Alcohol abuse	- Cigarette smoking
- Hemoglobinopathies (sickle cell)	- Gaucher's disease
- Coagulopathies	- Lupus
- Radiation	- Viral illnesses
- Organ transplantation	- Hyperlipidemia
- Cancer	- Pregnancy
- Occupation (miners/divers)	

Obtaining a thorough family history is essential as many of the less common disorders are inheritable.

Up to 20% of cases have no definable risk factor and are classified as idiopathic.

O

Perform physical exam
General: signs of systemic illness should be evaluated.
- For example, cushingoid features suggest hypercortisolism.

Lower extremity: pain and diminished active and passive ROM are found.
- Passive internal rotation is particularly painful.

- Complete evaluation of the contralateral hip is important as the rate of bilaterality ranges from 40% to 80%.

Obtain imaging studies of the hips
AP and frog-leg lateral plain film views should be obtained.
Negative x-rays do not mean that early osteonecrosis is not present.

- MRI is the most sensitive (80% to 100%) modality for detecting radiographically normal osteonecrosis.

- CT and bone scans can also be used but they are less sensitive.

Staging is based on MRI and radiographic findings and ranges from 0 (normal) to VI (advanced degenerative changes).

Send labs
If no history of any risk factors is present, a full medical workup should be performed by an internist.
A hematologist should also be consulted regarding specific blood tests and management.

Osteonecrosis of the femoral head
The diagnosis is made on the basis of the radiographic findings.
Etiology is not well understood.
- Osteonecrosis is the final common pathway of any series of disturbances in blood flow that leads to decreased femoral head blood flow and cell death.
- Microvascular coagulation disturbances lead to venous thrombosis and then retrograde arterial occlusion.
- It can occur anywhere in the body, but the hip is where it has received the most attention.

Occurs in 10,000 to 20,000 pts per year in the U.S.
Most common in pts 30–40 years old
Some authors suggest that most pts with idiopathic osteonecrosis have a subclinical coagulopathy.
Underlying medical conditions and causes should be evaluated and assessed.

No treatment or combination of treatments has been universally effective

Unchecked, the femoral head will progress to collapse in 80% of cases.

Treatments can be prophylactic or salvage/reconstructive.
- Degree of disease progression is the deciding factor.

Early Disease
Observation has proven mostly ineffective except in cases where lesions are small and outside major weight-bearing areas.
- Also indicated for pts who are poor surgical candidates.

Core decompression involves removing a 10 mm core of bone from the femoral head to decrease the intraosseous pressure.
- Associated with decreased pain, femoral head preservation, and delay in need for additional surgery.
- Effectiveness is limited in more advanced stages of disease.
- Can be combined with bone grafting; use of vascularized fibular grafts is gaining popularity and early results have been promising.

Osteotomies can be done to alter the area of the femoral head bearing the majority of weight-bearing forces.
- These are quite technically difficult, effectiveness is questionable, and further reconstructive surgery is made more difficult.

Late Disease
When advanced collapse and deformation of the femoral head occur, arthroplasty is usually warranted
Whether to perform hemiarthroplasty or a total hip replacement depends mainly on pt factors
- Older, less compliant pts do well with hemiarthroplasties
- Younger, more compliant pts should receive total joint replacements
- Very young and active pts should receive a hip arthrodesis due to the likelihood of the prosthesis wearing out and chronic pain developing

S **How did the injury occur?**
Most patella fractures are the result of a fall from height or direct blow.

Where did the injury occur?
This is particularly important with regards to open fractures or soft tissue injuries.

- Certain bacterial contaminants are more likely with exposure to soil (*Clostridium*) or fresh water (*Pseudomonas*).

Does the pt have any significant medical history?
Elderly, osteoporotic pts, diabetics, and smokers are more likely to have difficulty healing the fracture or surgical incision.

O **Perform physical exam**
Skin: evaluate for blisters, contusions, abrasions, obvious exposure of bone or joint cartilage.
- Both open fractures and open knee joints are surgical emergencies and cannot be missed!
Swelling: usually a large effusion is present due to marked hemarthrosis.
Palpation: a defect will be noted when the fracture is significantly displaced.
Neurovascular exam: though injuries to nerves and blood vessels are rare, a full exam should include function distal to the injury.
Knee extension: if the effusion is large or painful, it may be drained or injected with local anesthetic to determine extension.
- If the knee cannot be extended, the extensor mechanism is disrupted (patella fracture with retinacular tear).

- The ability to extend the knee does not mean that the patella is not fractured; if the retinaculum is intact, the knee can be extended!

Determine if the joint is open
If there is any question as to whether the fracture or joint is open, perform the *saline load test.*
- Place an 18-gauge needle in the knee joint.
- Inject 100 cc of sterile saline without removing the needle.
- If any fluid leaks out of the open wound, the joint is considered open.
- After performing the test, the fluid should be removed from the joint to decompress and relieve pain.

Obtain x-rays of the patella
Anteroposterior and lateral views are standard.
- Other views are difficult to obtain in a trauma setting.
- When possible, views of the contralateral knee should be used for comparison.
Pattern of the fracture, displacement, location of patella, and patella height are important.
- Amount of displacement (especially articular) dictates treatment.
- The patella should remain in the midline of the femoral sulcus.
- The ratio of patella length to patella tendon length ranges from 0.8 to 1.2 and is evaluated on the lateral view.
  - A ratio of less than 0.8 suggests rupture of the patella tendon.

Other studies are not usually needed to evaluate patella fractures
However, ultrasound and MRI are useful if rupture of the extensor mechanism is suspected.

Patella fracture

Common injury that was historically difficult to treat.

- Management formerly predominately nonoperative and associated with poor outcomes (nonunion, weakness).
- Early fixation failed frequently due to weakness of wire fixation.
- Patellectomy was also a treatment of choice.
  - Unfortunately, it is associated with extensor mechanism weakness and degenerative changes in the knee.
- Today outcomes are markedly improved due to understanding of biomechanics and fracture fixation.

 Determine whether the fracture requires surgery

If less than 3 mm of gapping is present with less than 2 mm of articular gapping, the fracture can be managed nonoperatively.

- Extension splinting or cylinder casts should be used for 4 wks.
- Pts may remain weight bearing as tolerated.
- Immediate physical therapy involving quad sets and straight leg raises.
  - No flexion of the knee is allowed at this time
- When x-rays reveal consolidation has begun, active motion and strengthening is started.
  - No passive range of motion should be initiated until the fracture is unequivocally healed.

Determine whether the fracture can be repaired

Various methods of fixation are commonly used to fix patella fractures, though most involve the use of tension band wiring constructs.

- Some fractures warrant partial or total patellectomy.
  - Most commonly, polar fractures (at the proximal or distal end of the patella), especially those that are comminuted, are managed with partial excision.
  - Severely comminuted fractures sometimes require total patellectomy.

After stable fixation, pts may actively flex their knee as early as one wk postoperatively and are immediately weight bearing as tolerated.

If the fixation is questionable, the knee should not be flexed until radiographic healing.

- However, isometric strengthening in full extension and weight bearing are initiated as tolerated.

S **Was there any traumatic event?**
A history of trauma, including whether a dislocation occurred, and the timing of injury must be obtained.

Describe the pain
Location, duration, intensity, radiation, aggravating and mitigating factors
- Can the pain be localized to a structure or is it diffuse?
- Are there feelings of instability?
- Is any particular activity associated with the pain?
  - Does it swell after any activities?

Does the pt have any systemic diseases?
Anterior knee pain can be seen with rheumatic disease, gout, Lyme disease.
- Is family history significant for rheumatic, crystalline, or autoimmune disease?

What pt factors may complicate treatment?
Consider whether workers' compensation or litigation is involved.
- Does the pt feel significant lifestyle or work limitations?
- Does the pt seem to want to get better?

O **Perform physical exam**
Begin with observation.
- Is there any obvious atrophy, swelling, or skin change?
- Is the gait normal or antalgic; is there a thrust?
- When the pt stands, are the knees in varus or valgus?
Palpation
- Areas of tenderness should be noted: ligaments, tendons, joint line, patella.
Assess range of motion (ROM).
- Is it full and painless when compared to the contralateral side?
  - Limitations in flexion must be aggressively treated.
  - Pain with motion may result from patellar articular injury.
- Is there catching or popping (seen with meniscal tears)?
- Is the pt excessively lax (hyperextends knee)?
  - If so, are other joints loose (generalized laxity)?
Note patella tracking.
- When the knee is flexed and extended, the patella should gently slide through the trochlea.
- If it sticks and jumps, malalignment (tracking) is suspected.
Can the patella be subluxed with the knee extended?
- Tight lateral structures or loose medial structures can cause maltracking.
- Is the pt apprehensive with manipulation of the patella?
  - Consistent with previous dislocations and instability

Obtain x-rays of the knee
Weight-bearing anteroposterior and lateral with Merchant views of both knees.
- Malalignment, fractures, degenerative changes are easily seen.
The Merchant view is taken with the knee flexed to 45 degrees and the x-ray tube is angled 30 degrees caudal from the femur.
- Normally, the patella rests centrally in the patella with no medial or lateral tilt, though judgment of tilt may be difficult.
- Apex of the patella should be medial to a line bisecting the trochlea.

Consider CT or MRI
CT taken in various degrees of flexion is excellent for diagnosing malalignment.
MRI is not as useful for evaluation of alignment but is helpful for evaluation of cartilage, ligamentous, and other soft tissue pathology.

Patellofemoral malalignment

Diagnosis is made on clinical and radiographic grounds.

Ensure that other causes of patellofemoral pain are not contributing (bursitis, patellar tendonitis, trauma, osteochondritis dissecans) prior to undertaking management.

If trauma is the cause, the medial retinaculum may have been compromised.

- Otherwise, the usual cause is a tight lateral patella retinaculum.

 Attempt conservative treatment first

NSAIDs with bracing and physical therapy may be effective for many pts.

- Aggressive strengthening of the vastus medialis obliquus allows compensation for excessively tight lateral retinaculum.
- Full range of motion is emphasized.
- Isokinetic exercises are generally avoided.

If physical therapy fails, consider surgery

Be certain of the diagnosis prior to surgery or the situation may get worse.

- Arthroscopic lateral release with debridement of chondral lesions has been effective in improving patella tilt.
    - The lateral patella retinaculum, vastus lateralis, and any adhesions divided after evaluation through the arthroscope reveals that the patella does not articulate with the medial trochlea by 40 degrees of knee flexion.
    - Subluxation is not improved, though, because no new stability is conferred.
- One out of 10 pts who have a lateral release develop medial knee pain due to chondromalacia of the medial patella facet.
- Aggressive physical therapy as before is initiated shortly after surgery.

If the lateral release fails, other surgeries may be required

Medial tibial tubercle realignment can be used to correct recurrent dislocations of the patella as well.

When significant degenerative changes are seen in the undersurface of the patella, tibial tubercle transfers will not be effective and patellectomy is required.

How did the injury occur?
As with adults, most pediatric ankle fractures are the result of indirect torsion.
- Children involved in high-energy trauma will warrant a more thorough assessment.

Does the story match the injury?
Child abuse or the possibility of a pathologic fracture (tumor) must be considered if the story does not match the injury.

Did the child have pain prior to the injury?
Benign and malignant tumor conditions are often painful prior to any injury and are not diagnosed until the fracture is seen.

- For example, fibrous cortical defects may be seen in up to one fourth of children.

Perform physical exam
General: ensure the pt is stable, especially in the case of a trauma.
- A full-body exam, including neck, pelvis, and extremities, should be performed.
Ankle: tenderness to palpation and swelling are usually obvious.
- Compartments should be examined to ensure they are soft.
- Pulses and capillary refill should be assessed and compared with that of the contralateral side.
  - If abnormal, arterial Doppler or formal angiography may be required.
- The neuromuscular exam is often difficult to perform in children.
  - If the child is unable to verify sensation to light touch, painful stimuli must be used.
- Investigate the integrity of skin and soft tissue.
  - Open fractures in children, like adults, are surgical emergencies.

Evaluate three x-ray views of the ankle
Pediatric x-rays are often difficult to interpret in the best of circumstances, and some fractures are quite discrete.

Stress views are usually not needed and may result in additional physeal injury.

- Stress views of the ankle should be obtained if a ligamentous injury is suspected.

Pediatric fractures involving the physis are classified using the Salter-Harris system
Type I: physeal separation injury
Type II: fracture line extends from physis through metaphysis
Type III: fracture line extends from physis through epiphysis
Type IV: fracture line extends through metaphysis and epiphysis
Type V: crush injury to physis

CT scans are not part of the initial workup
They are required for post-reduction evaluation of transitional fractures.

Transitional ankle fracture (Tillaux or Triplane)

Tillaux's fracture

These are Salter-Harris III fractures of the anterolateral distal tibia.

- Account for up to 5% of all pediatric ankle fractures.
- Mechanism of injury is usually supination-external rotation.

Anterior inferior tibiofibular ligament avulses an epiphyseal fragment.

- Occur in children aged 12–14 when the distal tibial physis is closing.

Triplane fracture

These are Salter-Harris IV fracture of the distal tibia with components in the sagittal, coronal, and frontal planes.

- Account for up to 7% of pediatric ankle fractures.
- Usually consist of a posterior metaphyseal fragment and a lateral epiphyseal fragment, though the epiphyseal fragment can also be medial.
- Epiphyseal and metaphyseal fragments are usually connected.
- Occur in children as young as 10; like Tillaux's fractures, pattern is the result of asymmetric physeal closure.

Attempt closed reduction and casting for Tillaux's fractures

The key is obtaining and maintaining an anatomic reduction of the intra-articular distal tibia.

- Non-displaced fractures can be placed in a long leg cast and kept non–bearing for 4 wks.
  - This is followed with 2 wks of using a short leg walking cast.
  - If any question of articular incongruity exists, obtain a CT scan.
- Reduce displaced fractures under sedation.
  - The foot is internally rotated and a mold is made in the cast over the fracture.
  - X-rays and CT are used to confirm that no more than 2 mm of intra-articular step-off is present.

Manage triplane fractures similarly

Casting of non-displaced fractures is performed as with Tillaux's fractures. Displaced fractures are reduced with sedation.

- Reduction method depends on epiphyseal fragment:
  - Lateral triplane fractures are internally rotated.
  - Medial triplane fractures are averted.
- Three- and four-part triplane fractures are less stable after closed reduction.
- After reduction, x-ray and CT are necessary to confirm adequacy (2 mm step-off).

If anatomic reduction cannot be obtained, perform open reduction

More than 2 mm of intra-articular step-off or physeal displacement warrants open reduction and internal fixation.

- Cannulated screw systems allow for accurate reduction and hardware placement.

Growth disturbance is rare

Occurs < 10% of the time with triplanes and markedly less with Tillaux's fractures.

S **How did the injury occur?**

Most pediatric femur fractures are the result of blunt trauma.

- Motor vehicle accidents and falls are common causes.
- Many are isolated injuries, but high-energy mechanisms are associated with injuries to spine, head, viscera, and extremities.

How old is the child?

The age of the child, as well as the pattern of fracture, determines the treatment.

Does the story fit the injury?

Nonaccidental femoral shaft injuries are unfortunately a common occurrence.

- Infants are most likely to sustain a nonaccidental injury.
- If abuse is even suspected, the treating physician is legally obligated to contact child protective services.

O **Perform physical exam**

ABCs and vital signs: especially with history of high-energy trauma, these are assessed first.

- Any abnormalities in the initial assessment should be immediately addressed by general trauma surgery.
- Head, chest, and abdominal exams should also be performed by the trauma team.

Secondary survey is where orthopedic assessment begins.

- Neck, pelvis, and other extremities should be fully evaluated for signs of pain, swelling, and neurovascular injury.

Affected leg: swelling, discoloration, shortening, rotation will be noted.

- The integrity of the skin and soft tissue envelope must be assessed to determine whether the fracture is open and a surgical emergency.
- The thigh and knee on the affected side should be evaluated for the presence of swelling or bruising, suggesting an associated injury (fracture or dislocation).
- Assess the neurovascular status and compartment tightness.

Obtain full radiographic series

The trauma surgeons will generally order the chest, pelvis, lateral C-spine, and "spot" injury films in the resuscitation bay.

- Required plain films for an isolated femoral shaft fracture include anteroposterior (AP) pelvis, AP and lateral femur, and AP and lateral knee.
  - Films should be taken before traction is applied.
  - With any fracture, it is essential to order films of the joint above and below the injury.
  - Fracture pattern, location, shortening, angulation, and displacement should all be noted.

Send labs and perform further studies and labs as dictated by the presence of any other injuries

Pediatric femoral shaft fracture
The most common major orthopedic injury in children.
70% of all femoral fractures in children are diaphyseal.
Peak occurrence is bimodal (ages 2 and 12).
Suspicion of abuse should be raised with younger children and stories that are not
consistent with the injury (spiral fractures, bilateral injuries, etc.).
Fracture malalignment should be no worse than 15 degrees of varus/valgus,
20 degrees of anterior posterior, and 30 degrees of malrotation in children aged
2–10 yrs.

- Children 2–10 will overgrow the femur by almost 1 cm after fracture (thus, a
  little shortening is acceptable and even beneficial).

 Plan and initiate treatment
Decisions on treatment must take many factors into account.
- Multiple injuries, child's age, cost, and fracture pattern and stability.

Treat children younger than 6 months with a Pavlik harness
Newborns may sustain femoral shaft fractures from difficult delivery or as a result of
a congenital abnormality (such as osteogenesis imperfecta)
- The harness allows for maintenance of alignment and is easy to manage
- Neonates have tremendous remodeling potential and can correct all but the
  most severe angular deformities over time

**Low-energy fractures in children aged 6 months to 6 yrs may be immediately
managed with a hip spica cast**
Apply the cast with the hip and knee both flexed to 90 degrees.
- Casts should not be applied until the pt is conscious and stable.
- Traction should precede casting when shortening of 2+ cm is present.
- Continue the cast for 6–8 wks.
- Surgical fixation is appropriate in cases of polytrauma.

Children older than 6 yrs can be treated in a variety of ways
In children up to age 10 yrs, 3 wks of traction with the knee and hip flexed to
90 degrees (90/90 traction) can be followed with application of a spica cast.
- The cast is not applied until early callus is visible on the x-ray and there is no
  tenderness at the fracture site.
External fixation may be used as a temporizing treatment to maintain reduction.
- Refracture rates and hardware complications are common, and it has fallen out
  of favor as a definitive management.
Flexible nails are commonly used.
- They allow for immediate partial weight bearing and can be easily removed.
- However, malalignment may occur if the fracture is unstable.
Rigid nails can be used in adolescents, as in adults.
- The nail is placed through the greater trochanter.

- The main risk is osteonecrosis of the femoral head, though this risk appears
  less with the trochanteric nail entry point versus the historic piriformis entry
  point.
Plates and screws carry intraoperative risks and offer little benefit over other
procedures.

S

How did the injury occur?
Up to 98% of these injuries are the result of a fall on an outstretched hand with the elbow hyperextended.
- The other most common mechanism is a fall onto a flexed elbow.

Does the child have pain anywhere else?
Most supracondylar humerus fractures are isolated injuries, but ipsilateral humeral shaft and both-bone forearm fractures do occur.

- 15% of pts with supracondylar humerus fractures have associated injuries.

Is the history consistent with the injury?

Up to 36% of supracondylar humerus fractures in children younger than 15 months are the result of abuse.

- In children older than 15 months, the abuse rate is 1%.

O

Perform physical exam
General: evaluate for any signs of trauma or injury at distant sites.
Arm: swelling is always present; the presence of deformity is variable.
- With type III fractures, an S-shaped deformity is noted.

Perform thorough neurovascular exam

Both median and radial nerve injuries are not uncommon.

- The vast majority of these are neurapraxias.
Injury to the brachial artery signifies a surgical emergency.
- Clinically, diminished pulses are noted distally.

Review x-rays of the elbow, humerus, and forearm
Two views of each are needed to evaluate the injury and rule out any other fracture.

Elbow fractures in children younger than 4 yrs are difficult to interpret
This is because the ossific nuclei of the distal humerus have not yet ossified.
- Supracondylar fractures may look similar to condylar and transphyseal fractures.

Assume that negative x-rays with a positive fat pad sign have a fracture
Even if a fracture cannot be seen on the x-ray, if the posterior fat pad is visible, an intracapsular fracture should be assumed present.

Supracondylar humerus fracture

Accounts for two thirds of hospital admissions for elbow fractures in children.
This injury accounts for 3.3% of all pediatric fractures.
Left side more frequently injured than right.
Almost always found in children, but also caused by high-energy trauma in adults
  • Almost 9 out of 10 occur in pts younger than 10 yrs old.
Peak incidence is in children 6–7 yrs old.
  • This is because maximal elbow flexibility and hyperextension are at that age.
    ◆ Hyperextension converts what would be an axial load to a bending force.

Classify fractures on the basis of displacement

Type I: a truly non-displaced fracture; seeing the fracture line may be difficult.
Type II: a variable amount of angulation may be present, but the posterior cortex
  remains intact.
Type III: complete displacement with no cortical contact.

Measure Baumann's angle

Baumann's angle is created by intersecting a line drawn through the long axis of the
  humerus and a line drawn along the growth plate of the lateral condyle on the
  anteroposterior view.
  • Normally, this angle is 72 degrees, and it is useful in determining the adequacy
    of reduction.

Cast non-displaced fractures

Type I fractures are associated with only minimal swelling and minimal risk of
  neurovascular injury.
  • Long arm cast in 90 degrees of flexion and neutral rotation should be applied.
  • X-rays should be evaluated in 1 wk to ensure that no displacement has occurred.
  • After 3 wks, the cast is discontinued and range of motion exercises are begun.
  • Return to full activity after 6 wks.

Closely scrutinize type II fractures to determine management

Type II fractures have an intact posterior cortex and are thus angulated but not
  translated.
  • Minimally displaced fractures can be reduced in the emergency room under
    fluoroscopy.
  • If adequate reduction is obtained, application of a long arm cast in flexion
    greater than 90 degrees should be performed to maintain stability.
    ◆ If significant swelling is present, close monitoring of neurovascular status is
      essential, especially if the arm is held in hyperflexion.
  • If adequate reduction cannot be obtained, if the fracture is unstable, or if
    significant swelling is present, surgical correction is required.
    ◆ Closed reduction should be attempted under anesthesia and two percuta-
      neous pins placed to hold the reduction.
    ◆ If swelling is too great to reduce the fracture under anesthesia, traction can
      be utilized until this resolves and pinning can be performed.
  • Pins and cast are maintained for 3–4 wks.

Fix Type III fractures operatively

Fractures are markedly displaced and unstable with a high risk of neurovascular injuries.
  • Closed reduction with pinning versus open reduction and internal fixation.

Complications are more common with displaced fractures and can be significant

Cubitus varus, neurovascular injuries, compartment syndrome, and loss of motion
can all occur.

S

What was the cause of the injury?
Pelvic ring fractures are usually the result of high-energy, blunt trauma.
- Insufficiency fractures in the pelvis can occur as the result of osteoporosis, irradiation, or tumors.
- The pattern of the fracture and associated injuries are associated with the activity at the time the injury was sustained.
  - Anteroposterior (AP) injuries are seen in motorcycle crashes and when pedestrians are struck by a car.
  - Lateral compression (LC) injuries are seen in car accidents.
  - Vertical shear injuries are seen in falls from heights and motorcycles.

When did the injury occur?
Significant bleeding can accompany pelvic fractures and close attention must be paid to the pt's mental status and level of anxiety in acute injuries.

- Changes in anxiety are seen early with significant blood loss, even prior to changes in vital signs.

O

Observe the pt
Any obvious deformity or injury must be evaluated.
- Most important are signs of either airway compromise or hemodynamic instability.
  - Changes in mental status and respiratory pattern or rate suggest closed head injury or significant fluid loss.
  - Aortic ruptures are eight times more common with a pelvic ring fracture than in cases of blunt trauma overall.

After the ABCs, perform a thorough physical exam
With open book fractures, the legs will be externally rotated.
Vertical shear injuries result in an apparent leg-length discrepancy.
Pull on the leg to evaluate for vertical pelvic movement.
Push on the iliac wings to determine whether there is any opening and closing.
Look for expanding hematomas suggestive of arterial injuries.
Ensure that the skin is intact.
- Open pelvis fractures are an emergency and associated with a mortality rate of up to 25%.
The genitals (including vaginal) and rectum require special attention.
- Bladder and urethral injuries are suggested by blood at the meatus.
- Rectal exam should assess for blood (possible visceral injury) and a ballotable prostate (consistent with urethral tear).
A thorough neurovascular exam of the lower extremities is essential.
- Traction injuries to nerves (especially the sciatic nerve in vertical shear injuries) and blood vessels are common, manifesting with changes in pulses, strength, and sensation.
Perform secondary survey of all four extremities and the spine.

Obtain x-rays of the pelvis
Three views of the pelvis are always required to evaluate a pelvic ring injury: AP, inlet, and outlet views.
- Classification is based on fracture pattern on plain films.
- Ensure there is no associated facture of the acetabulum, lumbar spine, or femur.

Obtain CT scan with reconstructions
Needed to further define the fracture pattern and plan management

Pelvic ring fracture

Most pelvic ring fractures can be classified using the system of Young and Burgess.
- AP injuries: three types
  - Type I: <2.5 cm of symphyseal diastasis (stable)
  - Type II: >2.5 cm of symphyseal diastasis with sacroiliac gapping
  - Type III: type II with sacroiliac disruption anterior and posterior
- LC injuries: three types
  - Type I: sacral impaction fracture with ipsilateral pubic rami fractures (stable)
  - Type II: type I with either iliac wing fracture or sacral crush
  - Type III: type II with contralateral sacroiliac disruption
- Vertical shear: force is directed perpendicular to supporting structures of pelvis.

Vertical stability is the essential feature to determine and is conferred by the integrity of the sacroiliac ligaments.

- As long as the posterior sacroiliac ligaments are intact, the pelvis will remain vertically stable (capable of tolerating at least partial weight bearing).

Associated injuries must be suspected with each fracture pattern

AP (especially II and III): pelvic vascular injuries, shock, sepsis

LC: brain and abdominal injuries

Vertical shear: brain, vascular, and abdominal injuries

P **Focus acute management on hemodynamic monitoring**

Unstable pts with open-book injuries can be placed in "butt binders" to decrease the pelvic volume and tamponade bleeding.
- These pts should be taken for angiography immediately followed by external fixation of the pelvis.

Surgical plan is based on stability

AP II fractures require only anterior plating.

AP III, LC II and III, and vertical shear injuries require anterior plating and posterior fixation because of the vertical instability.

AP I and LC I can be managed nonoperatively with weight bearing as tolerated.

S **What are the chief complaints?**
Peroneal tendon dysfunction ranges from irritation (tendonitis) with no instability to frank rupture of the tendons with severe pain and deformity.

- Pain is on posterolateral ankle, exacerbated by activity, and often associated with "popping."

Was there an acute injury or has the problem been progressing?
Often, peroneal tendon injuries are mistaken for simple ankle sprains; most severe insufficiency is the result of a long, degenerative process.
- Many pts have a history of multiple ankle sprains.
- Young athletic pts often recall a specific episode when they felt the tendon dislocate or sublux.

Is the pt active?
These injuries are more common in middle-aged, athletic individuals who engage in running and acceleration-deceleration sports.

O **Examine the pt**
Foot and ankle pain is often felt at a site away from the pathology because pts tend to favor the injured area.
- The entire foot and ankle should be examined regardless of the point of pain.
Does the pt have a normal gait?
- Often, the heel is fixed in varus with chronic tendon rupture.
- Determine whether any varus deformity is passively correctable.
Is the ankle swollen?
- Traumatic ruptures of the superior peroneal retinaculum swell significantly.
Palpate the posterior lateral ankle for tenderness.
- Tenderness will usually be exacerbated by resisted eversion.
- Tenderness anterior to the fibula is consistent with an ankle sprain.
Is ankle eversion weak?

- The peroneus brevis is the main evertor of the ankle.

Is the neurovascular exam normal?

- Symmetric weakness of eversion should alert the examiner to the possibility of Charcot-Marie-Tooth disease.

  - Charcot-Marie-Tooth is a hereditary degenerative disease that first affects the motor neurons in the intrinsic muscles of the foot, followed by the peroneus brevis muscle.
  - The hindfoot will often be in varus, the toes clawed, and painful callosities will be under the metatarsal heads.

Obtain x-rays of the foot and ankle
An avulsion fracture of the distal lateral fibular ridge is almost diagnostic of peroneal tendon subluxation/dislocation.

Consider MRI in chronic symptoms
Edema or fraying of the peroneal tendons can be seen on MRI and confirm the diagnosis

Peroneal tendon insufficiency

The peroneal tendons (longus and brevis) pass posterior to the fibula and are maintained in position by the superior peroneal retinaculum (SPR).

- It is rupture or attenuation of this retinaculum that initiates the cascade of tendon dysfunction.
- Forced inversion of the foot with plantar flexion is the usual mechanism in acute injuries.
- Most inactive adults with dysfunction have probably sustained repeated microtrauma to the retinaculum and tendons.
- Tendon subluxation and dislocation are the precursors to degeneration and tears of the peroneus brevis and, sometimes, the painful os peroneum syndrome.

Classification of insufficiency

Type I: tendonitis of the peroneal tendons with no frank subluxation or dislocation of the tendons
- Usually middle-aged adults with high activity level

Type II: SPR ruptured/attenuated, resulting in tendon subluxation or dislocation
- Peroneus brevis tendon may have a longitudinal tear or fraying along its edge where it rubs against the fibular groove.
- Generally young, athletic pts with history of an acute injury

Type III: degenerative tears of one or both peroneal tendons
- Heel will often be fixed in varus.

Treatment based on degree of insufficiency

Type I: generally respond to conservative treatment
- Walking cast or controlled active motion walker for 6–12 wks with oral NSAIDs
- If this fails, tenosynovectomy can be performed to debride the tendon.

Type II: debatable, with some surgeons advocating nonoperative treatment and others repair
- Nonoperative treatment consists of splinting then casting the ankle with the tendons in a reduced position for 6 wks.
  - This is followed with an aggressive physical therapy program emphasizing ankle strengthening and range of motion.

- Direct repair of the SPR (advocated for most competitive athletes) involves stretching the retinaculum and fixing it to the fibula sutures passed through drill holes.

- Longitudinal tears of the peroneus brevis should be suture repaired.

Type III: Repair of completely ruptured tendons is difficult; if one tendon is intact, the other is sutured to it.
- Often, complicated procedures involving osteotomies, ligament repairs, and tendon repairs are required for salvage.

S **How does the pt describe the pain?**
Pain is localized to the plantar heel and may extend through the midfoot.

- Usually worse in the morning

    - Improves with ambulation
    - Not associated with paresthesias

What risk factors does the pt have for plantar fasciitis?
Obtain a thorough history.
- Age (usually occurs in pts aged 40–70)
- Obesity
- Tight Achilles tendon (previously diagnosed)
- Pes palnus or cavus
- Repetitive activities
- Not associated with a traumatic event

Consider systemic medical problems
Plantar fasciitis can be bilateral in up to 30% of cases, but this raises the suspicion of systemic illnesses such as:
- Ankylosing spondylitis
- Reiter's syndrome
- Distal neuropathies

Develop a differential diagnosis for heel pain
This can be broad, but consider different groups of causes:
- Inflammatory arthropathies
- Tumors
- Infections
- Calcaneal stress fractures

O **Obtain radiographs of the foot**
Anteroposterior, lateral, and oblique views of the foot are mandatory.
- Special views of the heel (Harris) can also be obtained, particularly if there is a history of trauma.
CT, MRI, and bone scanning are usually not warranted.

- A CT or bone scan may be needed to evaluate for a calcaneal stress fracture.

Perform physical exam
General: look for signs of systemic illness (such as seronegative spondylo-arthropathies).
Skin: evaluate for swelling, erythema, and warmth.
- These are usually not seen in plantar fasciitis and suggest infection or trauma.
Foot/ankle: range of motion (ROM)

- Tight Achilles is associated with development of plantar fasciitis.

Tenderness to palpation on plantar calcaneus is found
- Pain in foot is worse with dorsiflexion and may extend distally.
Arch of the foot
- Is the foot flat or excessively arched?

Lab evaluation is unnecessary
The exception to this is if the diagnosis is questionable and the presence of infection or tumor is possible.

Plantar fasciitis
The diagnosis is made clinically.
Plantar fascia extends from calcaneus to base of metatarsophalangeal joints distally.
- It is an inelastic structure that stabilizes arch of foot during walking.
- Tensile forces are concentrated at calcaneal tuberosity.
  - This is where pain usually starts.

Etiology is undetermined
Pathologic evaluation suggests chronic stress.
- Microtears in plantar fascia in various stages of repair are seen.

- Pain is worse in morning because microadhesions form at night, which are ruptured with ambulation.

 Try conservative treatment first
Nonoperative treatment should be continued for a minimum of 6–12 months.
- Stretching and massage of plantar fascia origin
- ROM exercises for tight Achilles tendon
- Walking casts or controlled active motion boots
- Night splinting in neutral
- Ultrasound
- Steroid injections should be avoided.
  - Increased risk of plantar fascia rupture

90% of pts respond to nonoperative treatment.

If nonoperative treatment fails, limited release can be performed
Medial one third of plantar fascia can be released.

Excessive release weakens the longitudinal arch and causes chronic lateral foot pain.

Long-term results of surgical release lacking.

S How did the injury occur?

Most injuries to the posterior cruciate ligament (PCL) involve a posteriorly directed force on the tibia of the flexed knee.

- This often occurs in motor vehicle accidents or contact sporting events.
- Falling on a flexed knee is a common cause of PCL injury seen in football.
- Indirect causes, such as cutting and twisting, are also seen.
  - ◆ A higher likelihood of combined ligament injuries is encountered with these mechanisms.
- Determination of whether the injury is acute or chronic is important for management (discussed below).
- Isolated PCL injuries often present with limited pain in the knee.

O Perform physical exam

Begin with observation.

- Swelling may be noted but is often unimpressive in PCL injuries.
- Abrasions or bruises over the proximal tibia are suggestive of the mechanism.
- Is the pt able to walk with a normal gait?

Neurovascular exam is especially important in high-energy injuries.

- Sensation and motor function of the leg and foot are assessed.
- Color, capillary refill, and pulses should be compared to those on the contralateral side.
  - ◆ If any difference in vascular status is noted, an emergent angiogram should be obtained to evaluate the popliteal artery.
  - ◆ Vascular surgery should also be immediately consulted.

Range of motion may be normal in isolated PCL injuries but decreased if other ligaments are involved: always check the posterolateral corner.

Stability of anterior cruciate ligament (ACL) is assessed clinically with anterior drawer and Lachman tests.

Stability of medial collateral ligament (MCL) and lateral collateral ligament (LCL) are evaluated with valgus and varus stress tests at 0 and 30 degrees of flexion.

The PCL integrity is best determined with the posterior drawer test: flex the knee to 90 degrees and place the sole of the foot on the table. The proximal tibia is manually pushed posteriorly and the injury graded based on the motion.

- Grade 1: tibial plateau remains anterior to the medial femoral condyle
- Grade 2: tibial plateau is even with medial femoral condyle
- Grade 3: tibial plateau is pushed posterior to medial femoral condyle

Obtain x-rays to evaluate the injury

Begin with plain films of the knee: anteroposterior, lateral, tunnel, and sunrise views.

- These views show the presence of any fractures, avulsions, or degenerative joint disease changes.
- Pts with chronic PCL deficiency often have degenerative changes.

Consider MRI

MRI allows for visualization of the ligaments, cartilage, and meniscal structures of the knee and is also useful for confirming the presence of a complete injury.

Posterior Cruciate Ligament Injury

Injuries to the PCL were once thought to be rare, but recent studies show that up to 20% of knee ligament injuries involve the PCL.

- The PCL originates on the lateral border of the medial femoral condyle and inserts 1 cm inferior to the posterior rim of the tibia.
- It stretches from its anterolateral origin to its posteromedial insertion an average of 38 mm.
- The PCL can biomechanically be considered to consist of two bundles: an anterolateral band that is tight in flexion (and the more important band) and a posteromedial band that is tight is extension.
  - The reciprocal relationship between the bands of the PCL explains the difficulty in reconstructing the ligament with a single graft.
- The PCL serves as the primary restraint to posterior tibial translation.
  - The LCL and MCL are the key secondary restraints and become more important when the PCL is ruptured.
- It is also an important secondary restraint to external rotation.

 Decide whether the ligament requires fixation
Most isolated PCL injuries follow a benign course of recovery.

- Athletes with asymptomatic PCL injury are frequently found to have chronic PCL insufficiency.
- Several studies have documented that PCL tears that were treated with physical therapy have good functional outcomes.
  - Athletes who are able to maintain quadriceps and hamstring strength following a PCL injury tend to have full return to sport without limitation.
  - Residual laxity does not correlate with symptoms or poor function in cases of isolated PCL tears.
- The presence of a bony avulsion from the femoral origin or tibial insertion is an indication for reconstruction.
- Multiligamentous injuries should undergo reconstruction.
- Symptomatic chronic ruptures also fare poorly without surgery and are fixed.

Treat grade 1 and 2 injuries conservatively
Partial tears of the PCL should be conservatively managed in an aggressive manner.

- Brief splint immobilization with weight bearing to allow for pain relief and swelling is followed by aggressive physical therapy with an emphasis on quadriceps strengthening and range of motion exercises.
- Most athletes will return to sport within 1 month.

Restrict nonsurgical grade 3 injuries for longer
The knee should remain immobilized in extension for 4 wks to allow for healing of the anterolateral bundle of fibers prior to the initiation of physical therapy.

- Functional braces may be used to assist early return to activities.

S **What are the chief complaints?**

Locking, snapping, clicking, or clunking of the elbow, especially when it is being extended
- May also feel as though the elbow is sliding out of place

Does the pt have a history of elbow dislocations?
Most pts with posterolateral instability of the elbow have had one or more dislocations; with each subsequent dislocation, the force required is decreased.
- Pts will often relay that they are able to reduce their own dislocations.

Has there been any other injury to the elbow?
A fall on an outstretched hand, even if it does not result in a dislocation, can result in sprains of the collateral ligaments or fractures of the radial head and/or coronoid process and resultant instability.
- Childhood supracondylar humerus fractures (with resultant varus deformity), ligamentous laxity, and prior elbow surgery may also contribute to instability.

O **Perform physical exam**
Observation: look at the elbow.
- Usually appears normal, with no swelling or obvious deformity.
- May be in varus if history of childhood supracondylar fracture
Assess range of motion (ROM).
- Full and painless; if pt has generalized laxity, may hyperextend
Palpate elbow.
- Usually no areas of tenderness
Neurovascular exam
- No abnormalities are usually found
Assess stability
- No gross instability to varus or valgus stresses
- Posterolateral instability test is positive
  - Pt is supine, with shoulder flexed and forearm fully supinated and extended. The arm is then brought into flexion with a valgus load applied. Positive test result when the radial head dislocates, usually at 40 degrees, and clunks into place with extension.

Obtain radiographs of the elbow
Start with anteroposterior, lateral, and radial head views of the elbow
- Alignment as well as fractures (such as radial head and coronoid) can be seen
Stress views of the elbow in the posterolateral instability testing position show radial head subluxations.
The posterolateral instability test can be performed under fluoroscopy.
- With this, the elbow can be ranged and valgus and varus stresses performed with direct visualization of the joint motion.
CT and MRI are not indicated.

A **Posterolateral instability of the elbow**
Diagnosis is made on history and physical exam with radiographic confirmation.

- Insufficiency of the lateral ulna collateral ligament (LUCL) is thought to be the underlying cause of the instability.

All aspects of the injury must be established and managed.
- Coronoid and radial head fractures cannot be ignored.

Essentially, the bones of the forearm displace into external rotation and valgus with flexion of the elbow.
- The radial head subluxates posteriorly.

Anatomy
The lateral collateral ligament (LCL) complex consists of four components: the LCL, the LUCL, the accessory LCL, and the annular ligament.
- The essential structure for posterolateral stability is the LUCL since it is not only a varus stabilizer but also holds the radial head reduced.

Elbow stability is based on the integrity of the LCL, medial collateral ligament (MCL), and humeroulnar articulation.
- These are the primary elbow stabilizers and the elbow will remain stable as long as these structures are intact.
- The secondary stabilizers of the elbow are the radial head, capitellum, and origins of the common flexor and extensors.
- The minimal requirements for elbow stability are debatable.

P **Allow the pt to treat themselves if possible**
Avoidance of the aggravating activity is sometimes sufficient.
- Activities are performed with the elbow in flexion

Remember that conservative management usually fails
Braces and physical therapy may be attempted, but most pts are not satisfied with having a brace that must be used indefinitely

Surgically repair the injuries
The lateral ligamentous complex is reconstructed with the use of palmaris longus or cadaveric graft.
- The radial head, coronoid, and MCL complex may also require fixation.

- Medial complex insufficiency can be addressed with the lateral ligamentous reconstruction, but the graft must be passed circumferentially to correct both lesions.

Mobilize pts quickly postoperatively
A long arm splint is applied with the elbow flexed to 90 degrees and the forearm partially pronated.
- At 1 wk, a 30-degree extension block splint is applied for 6 wks, and then extension is increased by 10 degrees per week.
- Maintenance of ROM is the key factor for a highly functional recovery.

S **What are the chief complaints?**

Pain in the posterolateral aspect of the knee, instability, and difficulty climbing stairs or with cutting movements

- Pts with chronic posterolateral instability of the knee present with similar complaints.
- Up to 30% of pts with posterolateral instability of the knee have sensory or motor complaints in the leg related to peroneal nerve traction injuries.

How did the injury occur?
Usually, a specific traumatic event (2 out of 5 such injuries occur during sporting events)
- Mechanism usually involves hyperextension with both varus and torsional forces.
- A blow directed posterolaterally to the anteromedial tibia with an extended knee is the most common mechanism.
  - Indirect twisting injuries can also occur if the knee is extended, and rotation or abrupt deceleration (cutting) can also result in posterolateral instability of the knee.
- These mechanisms are associated with combined ligamentous injuries.

O **Perform physical exam**
Start with observation of the knee.
- Look for acute swelling, abrasions, or deformity.
  - Ecchymosis and swelling are seen after acute trauma.
  - Significant varus deformity may predispose to the development of or be a finding in posterolateral instability of the knee.
  - With ambulation, a varus thrust of the knee suggests lateral laxity.

Palpate the knee.
- Usually find tenderness over the lateral collateral ligament (LCL) or iliotibial band
Special tests are performed.
- Increased posterior tibial translation at 30 degrees of flexion = posterolateral instability of the knee.
  - If translation is increased at 30 and 90 degrees, posterior cruciate ligament (PCL) is also injured.
- Varus stress with knee flexed to 30 degrees, which results in joint gapping, is consistent with LCL injury.
  - If similar laxity is seen with full extension, injury to the cruciate ligaments (especially PCL) is likely.
- External rotation test: externally rotate ankle with knee flexed to 30 and 90 degrees.
  - Increased (compared to uninjured side) external rotation of the tibia at 30 degrees only suggests posterolateral instability of the knee; if also at 90 degrees, PCL is probably injured too.

Tests for anterior cruciate ligament (ACL), PCL, MCL, and menisci should also be performed.

Review plain x-rays of the knee
Start with upright anteroposterior and lateral and Merchant views.
- Avulsion of the proximal fibula or Gerdy's tubercle (where the iliotibial band inserts) may be seen.
- Avulsion of the lateral tibial plateau (capsular avulsion/Segond's sign) is consistent with an ACL tear.
- Weight-bearing films allow evaluation of overall limb alignment.
- Varus stress views can also be obtained to evaluate lateral structure integrity.

If the injury is clinically suspected, confirm with MRI
This also allows for evaluation of other soft tissue structures of the knee and planning of surgery.

Posterolateral rotatory instability
The posterolateral structures of the knee are a complicated series of ligaments and tendons that confer varus, translational (posterior), and rotational (external) stability.

- These structures act together with the PCL to maintain stability.
- The posterolateral knee can be divided into three layers: deep, middle, and superficial.
  - ◆ The deep layer is the most important, consisting of the LCL, the popliteus tendon, the lateral joint capsule, and arcuate and fabellofibular ligaments.
- The iliotibial band is a palpable structure on the anterolateral knee (part of the superficial layer) that is an important stabilizer of the lateral knee.
  - ◆ It is often spared in posterolateral injuries because it translates anteriorly in extension.

Up to 80% of injuries to the posterolateral knee are associated with injuries to other ligaments in both acute and chronic cases.

Treat pts with low demands and mild symptoms conservatively
Isolated posterolateral injuries have not been shown to cause functional limitations, even in competitive athletes, if symptoms are minimal.

- There may be a predisposition to early degenerative joint disease.

Treatment protocols usually involve short-term immobilization (less than 1 month) followed by aggressive rehabilitation.

- Rehabilitation focuses on quadriceps/hamstring strengthening and range of motion.
- Sport-specific activities are added as tolerated.

Early ligament reconstruction is advocated in combined or symptomatic injuries

Signs of instability resulting in functional limitations or associated injuries warrant reconstruction, preferably within 2 wks of injury.

- Any cruciate ligament or meniscal injury should be repaired concurrently.
- Varus malalignment, even if chronic, should also be addressed as this is associated with failure of posterolateral reconstruction.

Attempt primary repair of damaged posterolateral structures in acute injuries.

- In chronic cases, various allografts and autografts are used to reconstruct or augment the posterolateral anatomy.

S

What caused the injury?

Direct trauma to the arm, fall on an outstretched arm, and seizures can all result in fractures of the proximal humerus

- Seizures can also result in locked posterior dislocations of the shoulder

How old is the pt?

The energy required to cause the fracture in older pts is markedly less than in younger pts
- Higher energy trauma is associated with other injuries and more significant local damage

Does the pt have any other medical problems?

Consider a history of cancer or metabolic bone disease as a cause of pathologic fracture

- Osteoporosis is the most common factor associated with proximal humerus fractures

O

Perform physical exam

A history of high-energy trauma warrants primary evaluation by a general trauma surgeon prior to evaluation of the injured extremity

Skin: evaluate for bruising and integrity of the soft tissue envelope
- Open fractures of the proximal humerus are extremely rare but may be caused by extremely violent trauma
- Low-energy bullet wounds are not treated as open fractures

Neurologic exam: Full sensory and motor exam must be performed; every end nerve in the brachial plexus can be injured with violent proximal humerus fractures

- Most commonly are the axillary (up to 30% of proximal humerus fractures), suprascapular, and musculocutaneous nerves
    - Majority of these injuries are neurapraxias and resolve with 6 months

Vascular status: Decreased or asymmetric pulses, cyanosis, or paresthesias suggest possible axillary artery injury
- More common in the elderly due to arteriosclerosis
- If suspected, emergent Doppler and arteriography are indicated

High-energy injuries have been associated with chest wall and retroperitoneal penetration of the humerus

Obtain a trauma shoulder series of x-rays

This includes anteroposterior (AP), lateral, and scapular Y views
- In addition, two views of the humerus should be evaluated to rule out the rarely associated humeral shaft fracture
- If high-energy trauma is responsible for the injury, an AP view of the chest should also be obtained

Proximal humerus fracture
Accounts for 5% of all fractures and can occur at any age
Prevalence is increased in older individuals due to development of osteoporosis
  • In women, most fractures occur after menopause
The surgical neck of the humerus is the most common location of fracture
  • Three fourths of these occur in individuals older than 65 yrs

Classification is based on number of fracture fragments and displacement
Four parts of the proximal humerus are described: the articular surface, the greater
  and lesser tuberosities, and the humeral shaft
  • Fractures are considered displaced if any of the four major segments is separated
    by more than 1 cm or angulated more than 45 degrees
  • The greater tuberosity is considered displaced if it is separated by more than
    5 mm (3 mm in athletes)

Treat one-part fractures nonoperatively
Displacement of all fragments is none to minimal
  • These stable injuries involve minimal soft tissue injury and are best managed
    with early return to motion

Two-part fractures are often associated with dislocations
Isolated greater tuberosity fractures are seen with anterior dislocations whereas iso-
  lated lesser tuberosity fractures are seen with posterior dislocations
  • If displacement is minimal and there is no dislocation, sling with early return
    to motion is appropriate
  • Displaced fractures or those associated with irreducible dislocations must
    either be open reduced and fixed internally or close reduced and fixated with
    percutaneous pins
  • Anatomic neck fractures should be open reduced in younger pts and replaced
    with a prosthetic humeral head in the elderly

Open reduce and fix most three-part fractures
Young pts should almost always undergo open reduction internal fixation
Healthy elderly pts should undergo a hemiarthroplasty
  • Unhealthy elderly pts or those with social issues who are unlikely to comply
    with postoperative limitations can be treated with 3–4 wks of immobilization
    and early return to motion

Four-part fractures are often devastating injuries
Elderly pts who can tolerate a hemiarthroplasty should have one
Younger pts may be treated with open reduction and internal fixation, though satis-
  factory results are noted only about 50% of the time
  • Salvage procedure for young pts is hemiarthroplasty
  • Percutaneous fixation is an emerging technology for young pts with proximal
    humerus fractures

S   **What are the chief complaints?**

Insidious shoulder pain that is worsened by overhead activities with chronic tears
Weakness and pain with lifting

Usually no complaints of instability in older pts

Was there a traumatic event?
Rotator cuff tears (RCTs) in older individuals tend to be degenerative whereas
   younger pts often have sustained an acute injury.

   • Symptoms of an acute tear include severe pain and acute onset of shoulder
     weakness.

What is the pt's activity level?
Overhead athletes require more aggressive management than sedentary, older individuals and also have better functional outcomes.

O   **Perform physical exam**
Atrophy of the rotator cuff or periscapular muscles may be noted.
Decreased active range of motion with normal passive range of motion (ROM)
Neurovascular exam should be normal.
Specific tests that should be performed include:
   • Forward flexion to 170 degrees is normal.
   • External rotation is normally 30–60 degrees.
   • Internal rotation is normally up to the level of T6.
   • Impingement sign: passive flexion > 90 degrees resulting in pain

       ◆ Impingement test is relief of pain after subacromial injection of local
         anesthetic.

   • Hawkins' test: passive forward flexion with internal rotation; pain =
     impingement
   • Empty can test: resisted arm forward flexion at 90 degrees with the arm
     maximally pronated
       ◆ Pain or weakness suggests supraspinatus lesion.
   • Rubber can sign: resisted maximum external rotation with the arm slightly
     abducted
       ◆ Pain or weakness suggests infraspinatus lesion.
   • Lift-off test: place back of hand on buttocks and push out.
       ◆ Inability to do so suggests subscapularis lesion.
Other tests include various instability tests (apprehension, relocation), labral tests,
   biceps tests (Speed, Yerguson's), and Spurling's test.

     • Spurling's test involves lateral flexion and rotation of the neck with a slight
       axial load; assesses for a C-spine origin of the pain.

Obtain trauma shoulder series x-rays
Anteroposterior, scapula Y, and axillary views
Other special views can be used to evaluate for degenerative changes, impaction
   fractures, and osteolysis.
   • The supraspinatus outlet view is useful for determining acromial morphology
     (three types with type III being associated with impingement).
   • Osteophytes, calcification of the shoulder ligaments, and superior migration of
     the humeral head are seen with chronic RCTs.

Obtain MRI if clinical exam is consistent with RCT
Recall that the MRI is a confirmatory test because abnormal findings on scans do
   not always correlate with the presence of symptoms.

Impingement syndrome and/or RCT
The rotator cuff consists of 4 muscles: supraspinatus, infraspinatus, subscapularis, and teres minor.

- Supraspinatus tears are the most common, followed by combined supraspinatus and infraspinatus tears.

Most RCTs are the result of long-standing subacromial impingement on the supraspinatus tendon.

- Impingement is associated with a type III (or hooked) acromion that hangs down into the subacromial space and impinges on the tendon.
- With time, the tendon itself may be worn down and a full thickness tear may occur.
- Traumatic tears and those seen in overhead athletes (baseball pitchers, volleyball players) are seen as avulsions from the articular surface of the humeral head.

Subscapularis tears are sometimes seen after anterior shoulder dislocations and generally require primary repair or a tendon (usually pectoralis major) transfer.

Consider conservative management initially for RTC tears and impingement

60% will improve to minimal pain and normal ROM without surgery.

- Aggressive physical therapy focusing on RTC and periscapular muscle strengthening
- Oral NSAIDs
- Subacromial injections of steroids

If impingement does not resolve after 6 months of above and there is no cuff tear, consider subacromial decompression/acromioplasty.

Plan surgery if symptoms persist
ROM and pain generally improve with intervention.

- Most partial-thickness, degenerative tears are debrided.
- Full-thickness tears are repaired when possible with sutures or suture anchors.
- Tension on the repair is restricted for 3 months while the tendon is allowed to heal; gentle passive ROM and active-assisted ROM only for first 6 wks.

S

How did the injury occur?
Most scaphoid fractures are the result of a fall on a dorsiflexed wrist

When did the injury occur?
Many scaphoid fractures are initially dismissed as wrist sprains and not diagnosed until several weeks later

- A chronic injury resulting in a scaphoid nonunion presents with persistent pain, weakness of grip, and decreased range of motion

Where is the pain?
Pts complain about pain in the dorsoradial wrist
- Pain is worsened with use of the hand

How old is the pt?
Scaphoid fractures typically occur in younger, active adults
- Similar falls in older adults typically result in distal radius fractures instead

O

Examine the wrist
Snuffbox tenderness has classically been described as a finding
- However, the positive predictive value is poor because most pts with tenderness in the snuffbox do not have scaphoid fractures

The scaphoid compression test is performed by axially compressing the thumb toward the wrist

- This test has a high sensitivity and specificity for detecting scaphoid injuries

Obtain x-rays of the wrist
Up to 18 different radiographic views have been described to fully examine the wrist
- 97% of scaphoid injuries will be detected with only four views
  - Posteroanterior, lateral, and two oblique views are required

Remember initial radiographs may be negative in non-displaced fractures
X rays can be repeated in 2–3 wks to evaluate for early bony resorption seen in healing
- If a fracture is suspected, the pt should be immobilized until then

If suspected, consider MRI for detection of acute scaphoid fractures
MRI allows visualization of a fracture within 48 hrs of occurrence

- However, the modality is expensive and not always readily available

Consider CT scan to evaluate displacement and fracture pattern
These are also often useful in detecting acute scaphoid fractures missed on x-ray
- Thin sections should be obtained in the plane of the scaphoid

Acute scaphoid fracture
Scaphoid is the most commonly fractured carpal bone (about 80% of all carpal fractures)
- Main complications are avascular necrosis, malunion, or nonunion
  - Results in pain, instability, and degeneration changes of wrist
- Proximal pole and displaced fractures have a greater rate of healing complications

Anatomy of scaphoid is responsible for tenuous healing capacity
- Most of the scaphoid is covered with articular cartilage, leaving very little room for arterial penetration
- Blood supply is predominately distal to proximal; anatomic studies show that up to one third of scaphoids have little or no direct arterial penetration proximal to the wrist
- Poor blood supply is responsible for union taking up to 3 months longer in proximal pole scaphoid fractures and avascular necrosis occurring in up to 40% of cases

Classification of acute fractures is stable as opposed to unstable
Stable fractures include fractures of the tubercle and incomplete fractures through the wrist
- Unstable fractures include distal oblique fractures, complete fractures through the wrist, proximal pole fractures, and those associated with carpal dislocations

Treat non-displaced fractures nonoperatively
The fracture should be proven to be non-displaced by CT
- Various studies have suggested a variety of casting positions and lengths
- Most surgeons use a long arm thumb spica cast with the forearm and wrist in neutral for 6 wks
- A short arm thumb spica in the same position is then used for an additional 6 wks

Fix non-displaced fractures in athletes with hardware
One study showed a return to sport after an average of 6 wks with internal fixation of non-displaced fractures

Fix displaced fractures with hardware
Screws and K-wires are most commonly used; open reduction is usually required

Some surgeons recommend fixation of all fractures of the proximal pole
Reasons are the higher rates of nonunion and the need for anatomic reduction and prolonged immobilization

The optimal treatment for nonunions and malunions is prevention
Various osteotomies and osteoectomies are described, but results are variable
- The longer the duration of the malposition, the greater the degeneration and deformity that develop, and treatment becomes symptomatic

Consider treating avascular necrosis and nonunions with vascularized bone grafts
This procedure is most appropriate when no periscaphoid arthritis is present
- Long-term results (union rates) have been excellent

S **What are the main complaints?**

Severe pain in affected hip and often knee is chief complaint in slipped capital femoral epiphysis (SCFE).

- Usually follows a traumatic event
- With unstable slips, pt will be unable to bear weight, even with assistance.
- Often will recall a history of prodromal symptoms (previous pain)
- Often associated with a history of similar symptoms in the opposite hip

Review risk factors

Several risk factors for SCFE are established.

- Race (more common in blacks)
- Body habitus (obesity is a risk factor)
- Gender (more common in males)
- Age (usually ages 11–15)
- Family history
- Systemic disorders (hypothyroidism, renal osteodystrophy)

Consider differential diagnosis

The differential diagnosis for the limping child is enormous.

It is important to consider whether any systemic problem is contributing to the symptoms and the acuity of the problem.

- Fever, malaise, weight loss, and other constitutional complaints point away from a diagnosis of SCFE.
    - These suggest infection or tumor.

 Obtain radiographs

Anteroposterior and lateral views of the involved hip are required.

CT and MRI are rarely warranted in evaluation of a SCFE.

- MRI may be done to evaluate the viability of the physeal marrow and determine whether it has undergone necrosis.

Perform physical exam

General: evaluate habitus signs of physical maturity.

- SCFE is associated with obesity and endocrine abnormalities.

Lower extremity: assess for pain, range of motion (ROM), leg length, ability to bear weight.

- Usually diffuse tenderness at hip joint.
- Severe pain with active or passive ROM at the hip
- Often appreciable leg length discrepancy is notable.
- Ability to bear weight differentiates stable from unstable SCFE.
- Assess contralateral hip for silent slips (bilateral at least 25% of the time).

Obtain labs if warranted

Children younger than 10 yrs or older than 16 yrs should have endocrine workups.

Otherwise, routine lab assessment is not required.

Acute slipped femoral epiphysis
Disorder of proximal femoral epiphysis growth plate (the hypertrophic zone) resulting in slippage of the femoral head on the neck
- Functionally a Salter-Harris type I fracture
- High association with avascular necrosis of the femoral head

Most common hip disorder in adolescents (around 2 in 100,000)
Etiology poorly understood

- Mechanical factors are strongly suspected due to association with obesity.

Classify as acute or chronic and stable versus unstable
Chronic: prodromal symptoms present for more than 3 wks.
Acute stable: symptoms present for less than 3 wks but able to bear weight, with or without assistance.
Acute unstable: symptoms present for less than 3 wks but unable to bear weight, with or without assistance.
The significance of stability is in the prevalence of osteonecrosis.

- Osteonecrosis occurs in one half of pts with unstable slips but almost never in those with stable slips.

Radiographic classification schemes are based on percentage of slip and the head-shaft angle.

Plan for surgical treatment
Pts with unstable slips should be admitted and kept non–weight bearing until surgery can be performed.
- Some surgeons recommend gentle traction, but any manual reduction maneuvers should be avoided due to the increased rate of avascular necrosis.
- In the operating room, a single percutaneous pin should be utilized.
- The goal is to obtain growth arrest of the proximal femoral physis.
- Some surgeons recommend closed reduction and spica casting, others advocate open reduction with internal fixation.

Keep pts with stable slips or chronic slips non–weight bearing with crutches.
- The affected hip should then be pinned on an urgent basis.

Pinning of an asymptomatic contralateral hip is debatable.
- Rationale is to prevent the sequelae of chronic SCFE, which frequently develop in the contralateral side.

Complications are more common in unstable slips
Complications occur both from the SCFE and its management.
- Osteonecrosis
- Osteoarthritis (probably from altered anatomy and mechanics)
- Chondrolysis (destruction of femoral articular cartilage, which may result from thermal injury caused by drilling)
  - Presents with pain, decreased ROM, and joint space narrowing; results in early degenerative changes.

S Discuss history of symptoms

Children with a septic hip usually complain of severe pain, inability to walk, and marked discomfort with passive range of motion (PROM) of the affected hip.

- Pain is found in both the affected hip and the ipsilateral knee due to irritation of the obturator nerve.

Time of onset, any precipitating illnesses, previous trauma, and associated complaints should all be elicited.

- Onset of pain is generally very acute.
- History of recent viral illness or upper respiratory infection suggests another etiologic factor, such as transient synovitis of the hip (one of the most common causes of limping in young children).
- Associated complaints such as weight loss, night pain, and chronicity of symptoms suggest the possibility of malignancy.

Obtain detailed medical history

Beyond the acute event, a history of sickle cell disease or other hemoglobinopathies, metabolic abnormalities, neuromuscular disorders, malignancy, or hormonal disorders should be investigated.

 Check vital signs

Ensure that the child is hemodynamically stable and assess for fever.

Perform physical exam

Children with a septic hip refuse to walk on the affected side or bear weight.
Also exhibit severe pain with PROM of the hip and often complain of pain that radiates from the hip to the knee

Perform radiographic exam

Standard radiographs of the hip include the anteroposterior and frog-leg lateral.

- The joints above and below should always be imaged as well (knees and pelvis).
- Radiography has a poor sensitivity for detecting septic joints; an effusion or soft tissue swelling may be the only abnormality detected.

Ultrasound is often beneficial in detecting the presence of an effusion and in allowing aspiration of the joint fluid. If an effusion is present, fluid should be sent for analysis.

MRI and bone scans can also be used, but if the diagnosis is suspected, performing these tests wastes valuable time.

Send labs

CBC with differential, ESR, CRP, and basic metabolic profile should be sent, along with a synovial fluid analysis when aspirated.

- Synovial fluid aspirate with >50,000 WBC, glucose less than 50, elevated lactate, and/or bacteria is found in septic joints

Consider broad differential diagnosis for hip pain in a child

Infections, fractures, developmental abnormalities, tumors must all be ruled out

Septic hip
Diagnosis is confirmed by analysis of the synovial fluid aspirate.
Etiologic process is usually by hematogenous spread; traumatic inoculation or
contiguous spread of osteomyelitis can occur.
- Contiguous spread of osteomyelitis usually occurs in neonates, in whom
  transphyseal vessels are present allowing bacterial entrance into joints.

Distinguishing a septic hip from transient synovitis (virally mediated joint inflammation) is clinically difficult.
- Presence of three out of the following four: WBC > 12,000, ESR > 40, fever >
  101.5°F, and inability to bear weight indicates septic arthritis 90% of the time

Specific infectious organisms should be confirmed as soon as possible; different
bacteria are seen with children of different ages
- Neonates: *Staphylococcus,* group B *Streptococcus*
- 6 months–5 yrs: *Staphylococcus, Haemophilus influenzae*
- 5–12 yrs: *Staphylococcus aureus*
- 12+ yrs: S. *aureus, Neisseria gonorrhoeae*

 Treatment is early and aggressive

Children with septic hips must be emergently taken to the operating room for formal
irrigation and debridement.

Empiric antibiotics should be started immediately after cultures are taken and then
changed based on culture results; a first-generation cephalosporin or oxacillin is
usually adequate.
- IV antibiotics should be continued for 2 wks and followed with a 4-wk course
  of oral antibiotics, specific for the culture-proven bacteria.

Aggressive physical therapy is also immediately started to maintain range of motion
and return to activity.

Remember special considerations
Lumbar punctures should be performed in pts found to have *H. influenzae* due to
the increased risk of meningitis (*Haemophilus* flu is now rare due to the widespread
use of the vaccine).

N. gonorrhoeae usually elicits a synovial WBC of less than 50,000 cells/mL, does not
require surgical debridement, and responds to large doses of penicillin.

S **When did the injury occur?**
Acute dislocations can often be reduced without the need for general anesthesia whereas chronic dislocations must be treated in the operating room (OR).

Was this a traumatic event?
Pts with generalized ligamentous laxity or habitual dislocators (psychiatric issues) are not usually primarily treated with surgery.

Does the pt have a history of shoulder injuries/dislocations?
Recurrent dislocations are an indicator for surgical correction.

What position was the arm in at the time of injury?
Anterior dislocations (98%) occur through abduction, external rotation, and extension of the shoulder.

Does the pt have any other areas of pain?
It is important not to overlook any other injuries, especially with a painful, distracting dislocation.

What is the age of the pt?
Younger, athletic pts dislocate more often than older pts and are more likely to recurrently dislocate.
- This is due in part to higher risk activities undertaken by young pts, especially males.

Does the pt have loose joints or is he or she "double jointed?"
Pts with a history of generalized joint or ligamentous laxity often respond well to physical therapy.

Does the pt have any comorbidities that may preclude operative intervention or aggressive physical therapy?
If the pt has sustained significant trauma or has a poor general medical condition, surgery or aggressive physical therapy may have to be delayed or avoided.

 Observe the pt
In an anterior shoulder dislocation, several classic physical findings can be noted at rest:
- The arm is held abducted and internally rotated.
- The humeral head may be visible anteriorly.
- A subacromial sulcus may be visible posteriorly.

Perform a thorough physical exam
Inspect the skin to ensure it is intact.
Evaluate for an expanding hematoma in the axilla.
- Possible axillary artery injury
Assess the radial and ulna arterial pulses and compare to those of the contralateral side.
Assess sensation from the shoulder to the fingers.
- Evaluate for nerve injury (if present, likely a neurapraxia).
Assess motor function for a representative muscle from each nerve in the brachial plexus.
- Deltoid: axillary nerve; biceps: musculocutaneous nerve; wrist extensors: radial nerve; wrist flexors: median nerve; interosseous muscles: ulnar nerve
- ROM will be decreased, but it is essential to see that all muscles fire.

Obtain radiographs

A trauma shoulder series (anteroposterior, scapula Y, and axillary) view should be obtained for all shoulder injuries.

- Posterior dislocations are missed up to 70% of the time and can sometimes only be appreciated on an axillary view.

Additional views include the Stryker notch (view humeral head lesions) and the West Point (view glenoid lip fractures).

Anterior shoulder dislocation

This diagnosis is suspected on the basis of historical and clinical suspicion and confirmed by x-ray.

It is essential to determine whether any fractures are present in the humerus or glenoid.

Reduce immediately if possible

Isolated acute anterior shoulder dislocations can be reduced manually with proper relaxation (benzodiazepines, narcotics).

- After reduction, should be placed in a sling and swathe
- Shoulder should be immobilized for 3–4 wks in young pts and for 1–2 wks in older pts.
  - ◆ Elbow and wrist range-of-motion exercises should be started immediately.
  - ◆ Gentle shoulder exercises (Codman's) can be started after 2–3 wks of immobilization.

Suggested reduction techniques include the Stimson and the Kocher.

- The Hippocratic method should be used as a last resort due to the increased possibility of iatrogenic injury.

Plan for possible reduction in OR

Chronic dislocations, particularly in older individuals, should not be reduced in the emergency room due to the association with axillary artery injury.

- This has a 50% mortality rate.

Irreducible dislocations should be taken to the OR immediately.

Dislocations with humeral neck fractures should be open reduced in the OR.

Any pt with evidence of axillary artery injury should be taken to the OR immediately.

After any reduction, the neurovascular status of the pt should be reassessed.

Recurrent instability and associated fractures usually warrant operative fixation.

S **What are the complaints?**

Pts often complain of neck or back pain (usually acute in onset), worse at night and exacerbated by activity, and fevers

- Less common complaints include weight loss, dysphagia, and neurologic deficits.

What risk factors does the pt have for a spinal infection?

Spinal infections are more common in diabetics, transplant recipients, persons with rheumatoid arthritis, IV drug abusers, and those with any immunocompromised state (HIV, chronic steroid use).

- Diskitis is almost always seen in children; other spine infections are more common in adults.

O **Perform physical exam**

General: is the pt febrile, are the vital signs stable (rule out sepsis)?

Observation: is a spinal deformity visible?; look for paraspinal spasms

- Kyphosis is often seen in tuberculosis (TB).
- Paraspinal spasms are seen in 9 of 10 cases of vertebral osteomyelitis.
- Torticollis may be seen with a cervical abscess.

Range of motion of the neck or spine is limited and painful.

Assess for neurologic deficits.

- Uncommon (less than 10% of spinal infections) but may be sign of rapidly worsening condition (epidural abscess) requiring emergent surgery
- Meningitis can develop from direct spread of the infection.

Send labs

Several studies are useful in evaluation and following infections.

- CBC: white count elevated in 50% of acute vertebral osteomyelitis but less commonly in subacute infection, fungal infections, or disbitis
- ESR is usually elevated in spinal infections.
  - ◆ One fourth of TB infections of the spine will present with a normal ESR.
- CRP is elevated in acute infections and drops quickly with treatment.
- Blood cultures should be sent and held for 10 days but are often negative.

Image the affected area

Plain films of the spine are sent first, but these may appear normal for several weeks.

- Vertebral endplate destruction followed by collapse of the disk space is seen with pyogenic infections whereas TB tends to spare disk spaces.

MRI with gadolinium is the most sensitive and specific imaging modality for spinal infections and should be used for diagnosis and evaluation.

Technetium bone scanning used in conjunction with gallium scanning are almost as sensitive and specific in identifying spinal infections as MRI.

- Tagged white blood cell scans are not useful in evaluating spinal infections.

Obtain CT-guided biopsy to confirm diagnosis

Needed to rule out other diagnosis (such as tumor) and identify the infectious agent

Spinal Infection

Acute infections are those in which symptoms present for less than 3 wks, subacute 3 wks to 3 months, and chronic greater than 3 months.

Pyogenic Vertebral Osteomyelitis

Hematogenous seeding is most common mechanism, though direct inoculation and direct extension also may occur.

- Both the venous and arterial systems have been implicated as the highway through which seeding occurs.
- Usually a gram-positive organism (*Staphylococcus aureus* up to 75% of the time)
- Gram-negative bacteria are seen following genitourinary infections; anaerobes in diabetic pts.
- Other classic bugs: *Salmonella* in persons with sickle cell; *Pseudomonas* in IV drug abusers

Diskitis

Usually seen in children

- *S. aureus* is the most common organism.

Infection spread is hematogenous.

Tuberculosis

Infection of the spine is almost always due to hematogenous seeding.

Thoracic spine is most commonly affected, followed by lumbar and cervical.

Disk spaces are usually spared with TB infection.

Clinically, fungal spine infections look like TB and must be confirmed by biopsy.

Epidural Abscess

Usually associated with osteomyelitis or diskitis and spreads through direct extension of that other infection

- If it occurs without either of these, the infection is difficult to diagnose and will likely progress rapidly due to seeding of the bacteria into the epidural venous plexus.

Treatment depends on the type of infection

Pyogenic osteomyelitis is managed with a 6-wk course of IV antibiotics and followed with a course of variable duration of oral antibiotics.

- Molded braces are useful for pain relief and prevention of deformity.
- Surgery is used to drain large abscesses, manage neurologic deficits, correct deformity, and in cases where medical management fails.

Diskitis management is controversial; essentially all surgeons recommend bracing until symptoms resolve.

- The use of antibiotics is debated, though some studies show more rapid resolution of symptoms when IV antibiotics are used.

Tuberculosis is managed with 6 months of rifampin, ethambutol, pyrazinamide, and isoniazid.

- Indications for surgery are the same as those for pyogenic osteomyelitis.
- Similarly, fungal infections are managed with a 6-wk course of species-specific IV antifungal followed by an oral antifungal.

Epidural abscesses are almost always managed with emergent decompression followed by a 6-wk course of IV antibiotics.

S **Where is the pain?**
Talus fractures cause severe midfoot pain with inability to bear weight.

What was the mechanism of injury?
Forced dorsiflexion of the foot, as may occur in airplane crashes, is the primary force.

- The first thorough description of this injury was based on a study of 18 aviators who had crashed and sustained this injury (aviator's astragalus).
- Most commonly, a fall from a great height or a motor vehicle accident is the cause.

Does the pt have any subjective weakness, numbness, or back pain

Axial load injuries such as talus fractures are associated with thoracolumbar spine fractures (these are also common in calcaneus fractures).

O **Perform physical exam with trauma team**
Most of these injuries are high energy; many have associated injuries.
Observe the swelling of the foot and look for loss of normal skin creases.
Ensure that the compartments of the foot are soft and passive, and flexion/extension of the toes does not elicit severe pain.
- Rule out compartment syndrome.
Is the skin over the fracture site intact?
- 50% of type III fractures are open (classification discussed below).
- Even when the skin remains intact acutely, it is often under great tension and pressure from soft tissue swelling and fracture deformity.
- Failure to relieve this tension will result in skin necrosis and wound healing problems.
Are movement and sensation in the foot normal?

- Displaced fractures can lead to the neurovascular bundle from the posterior compartment (tibial nerve, posterior tibial artery, flexor tendons) becoming entrapped (especially types III and IV).
  - Decreased sensation in the plantar foot and fixed flexion of the toes suggests this may have occurred.
- Examine the thoracolumbar spine and remainder of the extremities.

Obtain x-rays of the foot and ankle
Anteroposterior, lateral, and oblique views of the foot and ankle and the Canale view
- The Canale view is an oblique view of the talar neck taken with the foot everted 15 degrees and the x-ray tube at a 75-degree angle from the cassette.
  - This view should be used to determine the initial displacement and adequacy of reduction of any talar neck fracture.

Obtain CT of the foot and ankle
2 mm cuts help delineate the fracture pattern and preoperatively plan.
- CT will also show any loose fragments in the joint or sinus tarsi that may cause pain if not removed.

Talar Neck fracture
Most common fracture of the talus, accounting for about 50%
One fifth of displaced talar neck fractures are open.
Mechanism shown in the lab is a forced dorsiflexion with ankle rotation.
The talus has a tenuous blood supply as it is covered by articular cartilage on 60% of
  its surface.

- Three main arteries supply the talus; maintenance of at least one is essential for
  the talus to remain viable.
- Posterior tibial is most important; also supplied by anterior tibial and perforating peroneal arteries.
- Talar neck is supplied by posterior tibial branches and artery of tarsal sinus
  (a branch of the perforating peroneal arteries).

Classification system used is Hawkins.
- I: Non-displaced fracture of the neck (1 mm or less displacement)
- II: Talar neck fracture with subtalar subluxation or dislocation
- III: Talar neck fracture with subtalar and tibiotalar displacement
- IV: Type III with talonavicular dislocation

Complications are common and increase with displacement.

- Osteonecrosis, degenerative joint disease, and malunion (usually varus) have
  been reported for all classes of talar neck fracture.
- While complications are rare with Hawkins I fractures, osteonecrosis and degenerative joint disease occur in more than half of Hawkins III and IV fractures.

Base treatment on fracture displacement
Type I: Non-displaced fractures can be treated with a non–weight-bearing cast until
  radiographic healing is evident (usually 6–8 wks)
- Frequent x-rays to ensure no displacement occurs must be obtained

Type II: Closed reduction should be performed in the emergency room with adequate sedation to reduce the tension on the soft tissues
- Unless soft tissue compromise is imminent, type II fractures are not surgical
  emergencies.
- However, even if the reduction appears acceptable, operative fixation is recommended for all type II fractures because maintaining the reduction is difficult
  and often fails

Types III and IV: Emergent open reduction is performed to reduce the pressure on
  the neurovascular bundle and thus potentially restore the talar blood supply.

Usually, perform fixation with two screws
Medial and lateral screws are passed from the talar head into the body or from the
  body into the head.
Postoperatively, a cast is placed and weight bearing is not allowed until radiographic
  healing is evident.
- After several weeks, the cast is removed and range of motion exercises initiated.

S **Obtain history of "bowlegs"**
How old is the child?

- Genu varum is physiologic until age 2 yrs.

- Beyond that age, bowlegs are abnormal.
- Infantile tibia vara can be diagnosed in children younger than 6 yrs old.

Has the deformity worsened?

- Genu varum should slowly progress to maximum genu valgum by 4 yrs (15 degrees varus to 10 degrees valgus).

How old was the child when he or she began walking?
- Tibia vara is associated with a younger age of walking.

Is there a family history of bowlegs?
- Consider the possibility of rickets or another metabolic abnormality.

Are both legs bowed?

- Infantile tibia vara is bilateral 80% of the time.

Consider risk factors for the development of infantile tibia vara
Several risk factors have been identified.
- Obesity
- Black race
- Early walking
- Females

O **Perform physical exam**
General: height and weight
- More common in obese children

Lower extremities: joint angles, range of motion (ROM), limb-to-body proportions
- Determine whether legs are in varus, valgus, or neutral.
- ROM abnormalities or excessive joint laxity suggests other etiologic factor(s).
- Disproportionate limbs suggest the possibility of a dwarfing condition.
- Tibial torsion should be assessed as it may predispose to tibia vara.

Obtain x-rays if appropriate
Routine x-rays are not warranted for children with physiologic genu varum.
Anteroposterior and lateral views of the knee and tibia should be obtained when tibia vara is suspected.

Consider systemic conditions
Several conditions are associated with the development of tibia vara.
- Vitamin D–resistant rickets
- Achondroplasia
- Renal osteodystrophy
- Osteogenesis imperfecta

Lab evaluation is usually unnecessary
A family history consistent with a metabolic or systemic abnormality may warrant specific tests.

Infantile Tibia Vara
Diagnosis is made on clinical and radiographic grounds.
Cause not established but likely related to repetitive and progressive physeal trauma
A less common late-onset form of tibia vara also exists.
- More often unilateral

- Demographics: obese, black, male teenagers

- Histology of both forms is the same
- Usually, a pre-existing varus deformity of the knees is present

Classification scheme used is that of Langenskiold
Staging is based on radiographs and considers changes in the medial physis and epiphysis of the tibia.
- Better outcomes are associated with lower stages.
- Interobserver reliability is variable with the staging system.

Normally, the metaphyseal-diaphyseal angle should be less than 11 degrees
- This is increased in tibia vara

 Consider that there is no consensus on management

Treatment is usually suggested for any pt in whom the metaphyseal-diaphyseal angle is >11 degrees.
- Some surgeons suggest observation in children younger than 24 months with metaphyseal-diaphyseal angles as great as 16 degrees.

Valgus unloading knee-ankle-foot orthoses are utilized in early infantile tibia vara.
- The brace is worn until the deformity is corrected and has a success rate of up to 80%.
- Bracing is most effective in children younger than 3 yrs.

Perform surgical correction if required
The goal of surgery is to restore a normal mechanical axis of the lower extremity.
- This is best achieved through a valgus-producing osteotomy of the tibia.

Surgery is most effective if performed in children younger than 4.
- Beyond that time, recurrence rates increase.
- More advanced disease (radiographically) is also associated with higher recurrence rates

In older children or those with advanced disease, other surgical procedures can be performed, but they are often technically difficult and have variable results. Consider the use of these procedures.
- Physeal bar resections
- Lateral proximal tibial hemiepiphysiodesis
- Combined tibial and femoral osteotomies

S **What caused the injury?**
Historically the result of pedestrians being hit by car

Most common causes now falls and motor vehicle accident

- Higher energy mechanisms associated with more severe and concomitant injuries

Complaints are consistent
- Severe knee pain
- Inability to bear weight
- Rarely changes in sensation distal to injury

Obtain general medical and social history
Advancing age is associated with different fracture patterns.

- Younger pts have a higher rate of ligamentous injuries.
- Older pts tend to have fractures with greater subchondral compression but no ligamentous injury.

Does the pt smoke?
- Smokers have more difficulty in healing fractures and incisions.

Does the pt have diabetes, vascular disease, or any immunocompromise?
- Pts with significant medical comorbidities may be best treated nonoperatively to avoid potential operative complications.

 Obtain radiographs of the affected leg
Trauma series of knee includes anteroposterior, lateral, two oblique, and 15-degree caudal views.

- Stress views to evaluate for possible ligamentous injury can be obtained after static x-rays have been reviewed.
- Comparison views of the contralateral knee can be utilized to evaluate for ligamentous injury if stress views cannot be obtained.

Views of the ipsilateral tibia-fibula and femur should be obtained.
Classification is based on plain films (Schatzker I–VI).
MRI is usually not needed acutely but can be used later to assess ligament and meniscal cartilage integrity

Obtain CT scan
CT scans with sagittal and coronal reconstructions are tremendously valuable for preoperative planning and determining which fractures are best managed operatively.

Perform physical exam
General: ensure stable vital signs
Lower extremity: assess from pelvis distal

- Soft tissue envelope should be evaluated to ensure the fracture is not open.
- Marked swelling usually noted in knee with decreased and painful range of motion (ROM).
- Neurovascular status should be evaluated and monitored.
  - If pulses are asymmetric or diminished, Doppler arterial studies should be performed.
- Compartment syndromes are rare but should be considered
  - Invasive measurement of compartment pressures may be required if the clinical exam is equivocal for compartment syndrome.

Obtain preoperative labs if indicated

Tibial plateau fracture
Diagnosis is radiographic
Ensure no associated or distant injuries are present (tibial plateau fractures are
 painful and can be distracting).
Any emergent issues (open injury, compartment syndrome, vascular injuries) must
 be identified.

Stabilize the fracture in the emergency room
Usually knee immobilizer or hinged knee brace is adequate.
- Pts should remain non–weight bearing with ice and elevation.

Consider emergencies
Open fractures (immediate debridement)
Compartment syndrome (immediate fasciotomies)
Vascular injuries (consult vascular service when identified)
Severely shortened or displaced fractures can be acutely managed with external
 fixation.

Plan for definitive management

Stable, non-displaced fractures can be managed nonoperatively.
- Hinged knee brace, isometric quadriceps exercises, and ROM exercises
- Weight bearing is restricted from none to partial for 8–12 wks.
- Unrestricted activities not allowed for 4–6 months.
- Pts who are poor surgical candidates can also be managed nonoperatively.
Surgical intervention gives best outcomes for unstable, displaced, or comminuted
 fractures; several options exist.
- Limited open reduction (small incisions with screw fixation)
- Open reduction (better when depressed or displaced fragments present)
- External fixation, including Ilizarov fixators (may use with open reduction
 internal fixation)
  ◆ Ilizarov fixation allows immediate weight bearing.
Importance of ligament repairs is questionable and not universally recommended.
Post op management focuses on protection of repair.
- Protect in hinged knee brace (except with Ilizarov)
- ROM exercises
- Limited weight bearing for 3 months

S **Obtain history of event**

Usually the result of high-energy mechanism, such as fall from height or motor vehicle accident

- Elderly or frail pts may sustain spinal injuries from lower energy events (slips and falls).

Is the pt short of breath or unresponsive?

Spine should be evaluated after stability of pt is ensured.

Where does the pt have pain?

Is there neck or back pain?

Is there pain in the extremities?

- Think about associated fractures.

Is there chest, abdominal, or pelvic pain?

- Think about cardiopulmonary or hollow or solid organ injury.
- These injuries are potentially life threatening and should be evaluated first.

Is the pt complaining of numbness or inability to move?

The presence of a neurologic deficit increases the necessity for a rapid full workup as therapeutic interventions must be performed in a timely manner, including possible emergent operation!

 Obtain vitals and ABCs, then observe and palpate

Hypotension may be the result of neurogenic shock due to loss of sympathetic tone.

- However, if hypotension is associated with tachycardia, concern for hypovolemic shock (from blood loss) should be raised.

Evaluation of skin and soft tissue after carefully log-rolling pt

- Open spine fractures are rare, but overlooking these injuries may lead to infection.

Palpate from occiput to sacrum.

- Feel for areas of crepitation, fluid collection, and tenderness, which suggest injury and warrant radiographic evaluation.

Perform a thorough neurologic exam

The exam for thoracolumbar spine trauma includes sensory testing for all dermatomes, lumbar and sacral nerve root function, and determination of reflexes.

- Reflexes tested should include superficial abdominal, cremasteric, patella tendon, Achilles tendon, Babinski, anal wink, and bulbocavernosus.

An accurate assessment of the neurologic status cannot be completed until spinal shock resolves.

- This occurs within 48 hrs almost 100% of the time.
- Spinal shock is basically flaccid paralysis due to disruption of the function of the cord.
- Resolution is confirmed by return of the bulbocavernosus reflex.

If a deficit is present, determine whether it is complete or incomplete

Complete injuries: total absence of sensory or motor function below the level of injury after spinal shock resolves (minimal recovery possible)

Incomplete injuries: some residual function exists distal to the level of injury

- Incomplete injuries have variable degrees of recovery, based on the anatomic location in the cord where the damage has occurred.

Obtain x-rays of the spine

Plain films of the entire spine should be obtained.

- Location and pattern of fractures determines treatment.
- If a single spine fracture is present, there is a 10% chance of a noncontiguous spine fracture being present.
- These injuries are missed a reported 50% of the time.

Obtain a CT scan of the spine

CT scan should be reviewed to detail osseous structures and deformity.

- Axial cuts with sagittal and coronal reconstructions delineate canal alignment and compromise.

If deficit present, obtain MRI of spine

MRI shows location and type (edema, hematoma) of cord injury.

Thoracolumbar spine injury

Classification is based on presence or absence (and type) of neurologic deficit and fracture pattern (compression, burst, seat-belt, and fracture dislocations)

Stability of fractures is based on the three-column classification of Denis

- Anterior: Anterior longitudinal ligament and anterior two thirds of disk and body
- Middle: Posterior longitudinal ligament and posterior one third of disk and body
- Posterior: Neural arch, interspinous and supraspinous ligaments, and ligamentum flavum
- If two columns are intact, the spine is stable.

Address injuries with a neurologic deficit immediately

Immobilize the injured spine with oscillating bed.

Administer IV methylprednisolone within 8 hrs to decrease secondary cord injury caused by ischemia and edema.

Perform surgical decompression to remove bony fragments or reduce dislocations.

The most emergent injuries are those with an incomplete but progressive deficit.

Reserve nonoperative treatment for stable fractures

These include all single column fractures (wedge, posterior element fractures).

Stability is based on deformity and likelihood of progression.

Plastic molded or cast orthoses are used for variable periods.

Plan surgery for unstable fractures or those with significant canal compromise

Decompressions and fusions should be performed on an urgent basis.

No consensus exists on the exact timing or indications for surgery.

S   **Does the pt have numbness or paresthesia in the hand?**

Ulnar tunnel syndrome may present with or without changes in sensation.

- If present, changes in sensation are found in the small finger and ulnar half of the ring finger.

Is there weakness in the hand?

Weakness may or may not be present.

- Pts will sometimes complain of weakened grip or difficulty working with tools.

Is the hand painful?

Pain is uncommon in cases of ulnar tunnel syndrome.

- The presence of pain should suggest the possibility of another etiologic factor, such as trauma or tenosynovitis.

What risk factors for ulnar tunnel syndrome does the pt have?

These are numerous and include:

- Previous trauma
- Diabetes
- Occupational exposure to vibration
- Inflammatory conditions (gout, rheumatoid arthritis)
- Alcohol abuse

 Perform physical exam

Hand: Full motor and sensory exam

- Hypothenar atrophy, decreased sensation, weakness of intrinsics may be seen.
  - ◆ Intrinsic weakness is a rare presenting sign in ulnar tunnel syndrome.
- Is there any deformity consistent with previous trauma (such as distal radius fracture)?
- Is there any tenderness to palpation?
  - ◆ Nonunited hook of hamate fractures may compress the ulnar nerve.

Obtain plain films to evaluate for bony causes

Distal radius and hook of hamate fractures are usually well visualized on plain x-rays of the hand.

- Carpal tunnel and oblique views of the wrist should be obtained.

Consider MRI to evaluate soft tissue causes of compression

These include ganglia and muscle anomalies.

CT is more sensitive than MRI or plain radiology for visualization of hook of hamate fractures

If a fracture is clinically suspected, obtain the CT scan.

Doppler ultrasound of the ulnar artery may also be diagnostic

Thrombosis or pseudoaneurysm of the ulnar artery may cause compression of the nerve.

Consider differential diagnosis

Similar symptoms can arise from a variety of causes

- Cubital tunnel syndrome
- Cervical radiculopathy
- Thoracic outlet syndrome

Ulnar tunnel syndrome
Diagnosis is clinical with confirmation by objective studies.

The elbow is the most common location of ulnar nerve entrapment.

Ulnar tunnel (or Guyan's canal) contains the ulnar nerve and artery and is defined by:
- Roof: volar carpal ligament
- Floor: transverse carpal ligament and pisohamate ligament
- Ulnar wall: hook of hamate
- Radial wall: pisiform and abductor digiti minimi

Location of entrapment determines whether symptoms are motor, sensory, or both.
- Zone 1: Begins at the edge of the palmar carpal ligament and is 3 cm in length.
  - Most likely causes of compression are ganglia or hook of hamate
  - Findings both sensory and motor deficits
- Zone 2: Surrounds deep motor branch of nerve.
  - Same causes as zone 1
  - Findings purely motor deficits
- Zone 3: Surrounds sensory branch of nerve.
  - Causes usually involve the ulnar artery (thrombosis most common).
  - Findings purely sensory deficits

 Attempt nonoperative treatment first
This includes the use of splints, NSAIDs, and activity modification.
- Avoidance of aggravating activities may be curative.

Perform surgery if conservative modalities fail
In addition, when a defined anatomic lesion is present (such as ganglion of thrombosis of the ulnar artery), the pathologic process should be addressed.
- If surgery is chosen, the entire length of the canal should be decompressed and the nerve visualized.

If the pt has carpal tunnel release, release of Guyon's canal is unnecessary

Release of the transverse carpal ligament (as in a carpal tunnel release) also decompresses the ulnar nerve.

Index